THE HEALING POWER OF HERBS

*The enlightened
person's guide to the
wonders of medicinal plants*

Michael T. Murray N.D.

Prima Publishing
P.O. Box 1260MM
Rocklin, CA 95677
(916) 726-0449

Editing by Robin Kelly
Typography by Janet Hansen, Alphatype
Production by Eve Strock, Bookman Productions
Cover design by Kirschner-Caroff Design
Illustrations by Cyndie C. H. Wooley

Prima Publishing
Rocklin, CA

Library of Congress Cataloging-in-Publication Data

Murray, Michael T.
    The healing power of herbs: the enlightened person's guide to the wonders of medicinal plants / by Michael T. Murray.
    p.   cm.
    Includes index.
    ISBN 1-55958-138-7 : $12.95
    1. Herbs—Therapeutic use—Encyclopedias.   I. Title
RM666.H33M865   1991
615'.321—dc20   91-18522
                                                                   CIP

92 93 94 95 96 RRD 10 9 8 7 6 5 4 3 2

Printed in the United States of America

TO GINA WITH LOVE

Contents

Acknowledgments

A special thanks to Dr. Joseph Pizzorno, president of John Bastyr College of Natural Health Sciences, and Terry Lemerond, president and founder of Enzymatic Therapy and Herbal Bio-Therapy. I truly appreciate their integrity and dedication to quality.

WARNING—DISCLAIMER

Foreword

I wish when I first began my journey into the wonders of natural medicine that a book like this had been available. For the intelligent layperson, there has long been a frustrating lack of access to accurate and reliable information about the many aspects of natural medicine. This dearth has been particularly evident in the area of botanical medicine: most of what has been available is anecdotal rehashing of material written more than 100 years ago.

Over the past 50 years, botanical medicines have been the subject of a tremendous amount of research, both in the United States and internationally. This research has resulted in the accumulation of a remarkable body of knowledge that repeatedly has shown, in both clinical and laboratory experimentation, the marvelous healing ability of botanical medicines. Yet little of this information has found its way into lay and professional publications, and few physicians are current in their knowledge of this important area. (Even naturopathic doctors—the only physicians formally trained in the use of botanical medicines—are not as aware of the science of herbal medicine as they should be.) I have often wondered why. I can only conclude—somewhat cynically, I must admit—that this is most likely due to several factors: (1) most of today's health care professionals are so enamored with the glitter of high-tech medicine that they lack interest in the less glamorous methods of mother nature, (2) the drug companies can make higher profits only by researching and promoting patentable (read chemically modified and synthesized) drugs, (3) doctors of natural medicine are so involved in their practices that they have not spent enough time reading the scientific literature, and (4) the publishers of general trade books often require their authors to write to a relatively uneducated audience. This book reaches beyond these constricting factors.

What makes Dr. Murray's work so unique and immensely valuable is his careful blending of concise and understandable clinical recommendations with thorough referencing from the peer-reviewed scientific literature. He has spent thousands of hours combing the international research on herbal medicines. When he makes a recommendation, it is both clinically relevant and scientifically proven.

While I respect and believe in the age-old wisdom of natural medicine and recognize that placebo-controlled scientific studies are not necessary to prove the efficacy of a botanical medicine that has been used for 1,000 years, that is no reason to ignore the wealth of information that researchers have gleaned. My belief is that the best information is that which combines and expands the best of clinical experience with applicable scientific research. That is what Dr. Murray has done here.

He has not avoided the challenge of writing to the intelligent reader in a manner that is truly informative. He uses and carefully defines technical terms as appropriate to further understanding while avoiding being too technical. The book can be used at one extreme as a simple guide by using the herbal formulas Dr. Murray has compiled, to the other extreme as a reference manual for the person who is seriously interested in herbal medicine and will pursue the comprehensive references provided at the end of each chapter.

This is a remarkably important and useful work.

Joseph E. Pizzorno, Jr. N.D.
President, John Bastyr College

Preface: A personal message

Many practitioners of botanical medicine are content to accept empirical evidence of a plant's therapeutic value and effectiveness, whereas others are intent on discovering whether the plant is truly effective and what its mechanism of action may be. I am in the latter category. What does botanical medicine mean to me? I cannot effectively express the feelings that have welled up inside me upon discovering the remarkable ways in which botanical medicines work. Humility, awe, wonder, joy, respect, and 1,000 similar emotions often overcome me as I discover the true beauty and harmony that exist in nature.

The more I learn about botanical medicine, the stronger is my faith in nature and naturopathic medicine. I not only want to share the information that I discover; I want to share the feelings. I hope this book will inspire you.

The bottom line that any practitioner or patient is after is the *result!* Botanical medicines must be used successfully if their use is to persist. Challenge yourself to study botanical medicine, and you will get results.

Live in good health, with passion and joy!

Michael T. Murray N.D.

INTRODUCTION

Botanical medicine— a modern perspective

$\mathbf{A}$re herbs effective medicinal agents, or is their use merely a reflection of folklore, outdated theories, and myth? Uninformed persons generally think of herbs as ineffective medicines used prior to the advent of more effective synthetic drugs. Others think of herbs simply as sources of compounds to isolate and then market as drugs. But to some, herbs and crude plant extracts are effective medicines to be respected and appreciated.

For many of the people of the world, botanical medicines are the only therapeutic agents available. It is difficult to assess accurately the extent to which plants are used as medicines throughout the world, but the World Health Organization has estimated that 80% of the world's population may rely on "traditional" medicines for their primary health care needs. Because botanical medicine is the major part of traditional therapies, it can be safely stated that the majority of the people of the world rely on plants as medicines.

The study of botanical medicine spans the breadth of pharmacology, which is the study of the history, source, physical and chemical properties, mechanisms of action, absorption, distribution, biotransformation, excretion, and therapeutic uses of "drugs." In many respects, the pharmacological investigation of botanical medicine is just beginning. This book is full of examples of herbs whose historical uses are being justified by new investigations into their pharmacology.

Although botanical medicine has existed since the dawn of time, our knowledge of how plants actually affect human physiology remains largely a mystery. Many individuals formulate their view of botanical medicine based on opinion, philosophy, and ideology. This chapter seeks to uncloud some of the mystery of botanical medicine and allow the reader to formulate an educated and informed view of botanical medicine. The past, as well as the future, of botanical medicines are discussed. For the study of botanical medicine to evolve, there must be a continuation of the tradition of herbal medicine within the context of continued scientific investigation.

Pharmaceutical use of plant medicines

Many plants certainly contain compounds that have a high degree of pharmacological activity. It is generally unknown that for the past 25 years, about 25% of all prescription drugs in the United States have contained active constituents obtained from plants. In 1980 alone, Americans paid more than $8 billion for prescription drugs in which the active principles were obtained from plants.

One of the great fallacies promoted by the U.S. medical establishment is that there is no firm scientific evidence for the use of many natural therapies, including botanical medicine. This assertion is simply not true. In fact, during the last 10 to 20 years there has been a literal explosion of information concerning plants, crude plant extracts, and nutritional substances as medicinal agents.

Scientific and medical technologies are now available to understand and properly evaluate botanical medicines. Thirty years ago it was impossible to determine exactly how herbs promote their healing effects because science had not advanced to a sufficient level of understanding. This point is well illustrated by the example of scientists' understanding of how aspirin works; the main mechanism of action responsible for aspirin's anti-inflammatory effect was not understood until the early 1970s, and its mechanism of action for pain relief has yet to be fully understood.

Since the mechanism of therapeutic action of a particular herb was not fully understood previously, many effective plant medicines were erroneously labeled as possessing no pharmacological activity. But now, researchers equipped with greater understanding and more sophisticated technology are rediscovering the wonder of plants as medicinal agents. Much of the increased understanding is, ironically, a result of synthetic drug research.

For example, one of the latest classes of so-called "wonder drugs" are the calcium-channel blocking drugs. These drugs block the entry of calcium into smooth muscle cells, thereby inhibiting contraction and promoting muscular relaxation. Calcium-channel blocking drugs are currently being used in the treatment of high blood pressure, angina, asthma, and other conditions associated with smooth muscle contraction. In many ways, they represent the highest stage of modern drug pharmacy sophistication. After calcium-channel drugs became better understood, it was discovered that many herbs contain components that possess calcium-channel blocking activity. In most cases, the historical use of these herbs correspond to their calcium-channel blocking activity.

In addition to possessing currently understood pharmacological activity, many herbs possess pharmacological actions that are not at all consistent with modern pharmacological understanding. For example, many herbs appear to impact homeostatic control mechanisms to aid normalization of many of the body's processes. When there is a hyperstate, the herb will have a lowering effect, and when there is a hypostate, it will have a heightening effect. This action is totally baffling to orthodox pharmacologists but not to experienced herbalists who have used terms such as *alterative, amphiteric, adaptogenic,* or *tonic* to describe this effect.

The advantages of botanical medicines

People often ask, "What advantages do botanical medicines have over synthetic drugs?" As a rule, botanical preparations are less toxic than their synthetic counterparts and offer less risk of side effects. Obviously, there are exceptions to this rule. In addition, the mechanism of action of an herb is often to correct the underlying cause. In contrast, a synthetic drug is often designed to alleviate the symptom or effect without addressing the underlying cause. It has also been demonstrated with many plants that the whole plant or crude extract is much more effective than isolated constituents.

Botanical medicine will certainly play a major role in the medicine of the future. As modern medicine gains greater knowledge and understanding about health and disease, it is adopting therapies that are more natural and less toxic. Life-style modification, stress reduction, exercise, meditation, dietary changes, and many other traditional naturopathic therapies are becoming much more popular in standard medical circles, illustrating the paradigm shift that is occurring in medicine. What was once scoffed at is now becoming generally accepted as effective alternatives. In fact, in most instances natural alternatives offer significant benefit over standard medical practices.

There is a growing appreciation of the harmonious healing properties that botanical medicine possess, particularly in Europe and Asia. Americans too are becoming more aware of the tremendous medicinal value of herbs. Without a doubt, the medicine of the future will make good use of botanical medicine: the medicine of the past will be the medicine of the future.

The difference will be a result of the growing sophistication of botanical medicine. With the continuing advancement in science and technology, there has been a great improvement in the quality of botanical medicines available. Improvements in cultivation techniques, coupled with improvements in quality control and standardization of potency, will continue to increase the effectiveness of botanical medicines.

Herbal medicine from prehistoric times to the 21st century—a brief history

Introduction

Plants have been used as medicines since the dawn of animal life. The initial use of plants as medicines by humans is thought to be a result of "instinctive" dowsing. Animals in the wild still provide evidence that this phenomenon occurs; animals will eat those plants that will heal them and avoid those plants that will do them harm. Presumably, humans also possessed this instinct at one time. Eventually, people began to analyze and cultivate what they knew about plant medicines. As civilizations developed, medicine men and women transmitted the information on herbs to their successors. Before the advent of written language, this information was handed down by verbal and experiential means.

It was commonly believed that plants had been signed by the "creator" with some visible or other clue that would indicate its therapeutic use. This concept is commonly referred to as "The Doctrine of Signatures." Examples of this doctrine include ginseng (*Panax ginseng*), whose root bears strong resemblance to a human figure and whose general use is as a tonic; blue cohosh (*Caulophyllum thalictroides*), whose branches are arranged like limbs in spasm, indicating its usefulness in the treatment of muscular spasm; bloodroot (*Sanguinaria canadensis*), whose roots and sap are a beautiful blood color, corresponding to its traditional use as a "blood purifier"; lobelia (*Lobelia inflata*), whose flowers are shaped like a stomach, corresponding to its emetic qualities; and goldenseal (*Hydrastis canadensis*), whose yellow-green root signifies its use in jaundice as well as infectious processes. All these uses have been confirmed by recent research.

With the development of written language, *materia medicas* (books containing prescribing notes on herbs) became the vehicle for passing information on the medicinal use of herbs to future herbalists. *Materia medicas* were recorded in ancient China, Babylon, Egypt, India, Greece, and other parts of the world. From these *materia medicas*, it is obvious that botanical medicines were highly respected in ancient times.

Galen's influence

There was no system, rules, or classification to Western herbal *materia medicas* until the first century A.D., when Galen, a Roman physician, established his system of rules and classification. Galen's classification was based on Hippocratic medicine—i.e., balance of the four humours: blood, bile, phlegm, and choler.

Each plant was evaluated and discussed in its relation to Hippocratic medicine. Although using Hippocratic principles, Galen in essence used this system to construct his own elaborate and rigid system of medicine. Galen's work signified the beginning of a clear division between the professional physician and the traditional healer. Only the well educated could understand Galen's system, but even with the best schooling it remained a mystery to many. All challenges therefore were effectively squelched by dogma.

Galen's system effectively paralyzed European medical thinking for 1,500 years. Perhaps if the Roman Empire had continued to flourish, someone would have surfaced to rival Galen. Instead, Galenical medicine dominated the Middle Ages. The "professional" physician, confident in a superior knowledge, attempted to hasten recovery by bloodletting, purging, and administering exotic medicines. This was in direct contrast to the traditional healer's patient use of traditional herbs and the tremendous faith in the healing power of nature.

The Black Plague and syphilis

Although Galenical medicine dominated the Middle Ages, herbal medicine was still deeply entrenched in European culture. The plague of 1348 A.D. may have been the beginning of change in medical thought because conventional medicine was totally useless. Nearly one-third of Europe died as a result of this plague, so the public began to lose faith in Galenical medicine.

Nearly 150 years later, another blow was dealt to Galenical medicine when syphilis became the major medical problem. Unlike the Black Plague, syphilis enabled its victims to survive longer, giving physicians more time to experiment with treatments. At this time perhaps the greatest hoax in the history of medicine began. Mercury became the standard medical treatment for syphilis, although even Galen thought mercury too poisonous to use.

Syphilis did, however, open the door for the use of some new herbs from the Americas. A French physician, Nicholas Monardes, published a comprehensive account of sarsaparilla and several other "new" drugs in the treatment of syphilis in 1574. Many Europeans at the time believed that syphilis had come to Europe from the West Indies with Columbus' sailors, and since there was a general belief that whatever disease was native to a country might be cured by the medicinal herbs growing in that region, it was only natural for sarsaparilla to become a very popular remedy. Since at that time the standard treatment of syphilis was the use of mercury, which often resulted in greater morbidity than did the disease itself, sarsaparilla was a welcome alternative. Despite receiving a favorable response initially, Monardes' sarsaparilla cure eventually lost favor, probably due to other components in the cure—specifically, patients were confined to a warm room for 30 days, and for the following 40 days were to abstain from both wine and sexual intercourse.

Although the public popularity of sarsaparilla waned, it continued to be used in the treatment of syphilis. During military operations in Portugal in 1812, a British Inspector General of Hospitals noted that the Portuguese soldiers suffering from syphilis who used sarsaparilla recovered much faster and more completely than their British counterparts who were treated with mercury.

The Chinese also used sarsaparilla in the treatment of syphilis. Later, clinical observations in China demonstrated, through blood tests, that sarsaparilla is effective in about 90% of cases of acute syphilis and about 50% of cases of chronic syphilis.

Although sarsaparilla was clearly more beneficial than mercury in the treatment of syphilis, mercury became established as the standard treatment for more than four and a half centuries. This treatment was indeed a colossal hoax. Mercury represented a new kind of medicine, one formulated and prepared in a laboratory using the new techniques of chemistry. It helped prepare the way for future drugs at the expense of herbal medicines.

Challenges to Galenical medicine

The 1500s also saw a strong challenge to Galenical medicine from within the traditional circles. Paracelsus, an alchemist who believed strongly in the Doctrine of Signatures, was responsible for founding modern pharmaceutical medicine. He probably is best remembered for the development of laudanum (tincture of opium). After Paracelsus, Galenical preparations and treatments fell greatly out of favor.

In public circles, herbal medicine was regaining some respect as well. In the early 1600s, Culpepper, an English pharmacist, published his book titled *The English Physician*. Instead of requiring patients to purchase expensive exotic or imported drugs, Culpepper recommended the herbs his clients and readers had growing in their own backyards. Although Culpepper's herbal is based on astrological rationalizations, it reinforced a strong English tradition of domestic herbal medicine. This came at a time when professional physicians were beginning to become contemptuous of herbal medicine.

Meanwhile, during the 1600s and 1700s, herbs used traditionally by Native Americans were becoming quite popular with colonists, especially in the treatment of malaria and scurvy. Botanical medicine continued to gain respect in the late 1700s, as exemplified by William Withering's classic description of digitalis. However, mercury, bleeding, and purging were still the standard medical treatments. These standard treatments were epitomized by George Washington's death from complications incurred during treatment of a sore throat (i.e., he was bled to death).

The Thomsonian and Eclectic movements

During the early 1800s, standard medicine may have been ready to return to traditional herbal remedies, but then came the Thomsonian movement. Samuel Thomson (1769–1843) patented a system of botanical medicine that, in 1839, claimed over 3 million faithful followers. Although Thomson brought back to medicine the Hippocratic idea of *vis medicatrix naturae* and gained widespread public support for the use of herbal medicine, the Thomsonian movement was probably detrimental to medical reform.

Thomsonianism was founded on ignorance, prejudice, and dogma. Thomsonians insisted that all medical knowledge was complete and could be found in Samuel Thomson's works. These and other claims roused scorn, indignation, rage, and resentment in the average North American doctor. In essence, Thomson's treatments often were as harsh as the standard treatments of the times.

During the 1800s, the Eclectic movement attempted to bridge the gaps between standard medical thought, Thomsonianism, and traditional herbal medicines. Rather than attack the existing medical system, the Eclectic movement sought to bring about reform by educating physicians about the use of herbal medicines. Several Eclectic medical colleges were established and, for a while, it appeared that the Eclectic movement was making headway in its attempt to reform the medical system from within.

The movement, however, eventually failed. Several factors were probably responsible for the failure of the Eclectic movement: a split in the ranks diluted the movement; physicians generally discarded harsh treatments such as mercury, calomel, and bloodletting, due to a decrease in infectious disease as a result of improved sanitation and hygiene; and, perhaps the most important reason, the movement failed to sustain a quality medical school.

The Flexner report on medical education in 1910 spelled doom for the eclectics: by 1920, seven of the eight schools that existed prior to the report had closed, with the last school closing in 1938. Meanwhile, the standard medical schools, aided by the Rockefeller Foundation, flourished, promoting the growth of the modern pharmaceutical industry and the current near-monopoly of the medical profession.

The growth of the pharmaceutical industry

Since a plant cannot be patented, very little research has been done this century on plants as medicinal agents by the large American pharmaceutical firms. Instead, researchers screen plants for biological activity and then isolate the so-called "active" constituents. Much to the dismay of the researchers, the isolated constituent has been found in many instances to be less biologically active than the crude herb. Since the crude herb provides no economic reward to the pharmaceutical firm in the United States, the crude herb or extract never reaches the marketplace. In contrast, European policies on herbal medicines makes it economically feasible for companies to research and develop crude phytopharmaceuticals.

Another problem of herbal medicine in the United States has been the lack of standardization. The herb that best exemplifies this dilemma is digitalis. One batch of crude digitalis might have an extremely low level of active constituents, making the crude herb ineffective, while the next batch might be unusually high in active constituents, resulting in toxicity or even death when the standard amount is used. The lack of standardization makes it easier for U.S. pharmaceutical firms to rationalize their economic need to isolate, purify, and chemically modify the active constituents of digitalis so they can market these compounds as drugs. The problem with using the pure active constituent is that the safe dosage range is smaller: digitalis toxicity and death has increased dramatically as a result of purification. Toxicity is less of a factor when using the crude herb because overconsumption of potentially toxic doses results in vomiting or diarrhea, thus avoiding the heart disturbance and fatal effects that may occur with pure digitalis cardiac glycoside drugs.

Fortunately, several European and Asian pharmaceutical firms began specializing in phytopharmaceuticals in the early part of the 20th century. These companies have played a prominent role in researching, developing, and promoting botanical medicines.

Research demonstrates that crude extracts often have greater therapeutic benefit than the isolated active constituent. This fact has been known for quite some time in other parts of the world, but in this country isolated plant drugs are still thought of as having the greatest therapeutic effect. This myth is gradually being eroded as our knowledge of botanical medicines increases. If current standardization techniques had been available earlier in this century, possibly the majority of our current prescription drugs would now be crude herbal extracts instead of isolated and modified active constituents.

Improvements in the production of botanical medicines

During the past 60 years, there have been tremendous improvements in extraction, analytical, isolation, and cultivation techniques as well as specific pharmacologic knowledge of botanical medicines, resulting in considerable improvements in quality control. Throughout the entire production of standardized botanical extracts, quality control and good manufacturing procedures are employed, including microscopic, physical, chemical/physical, and biological analyses. The European Council has set forth very strict guidelines for acceptable levels of impurities, including parasites (bacterial counts), pesticides, residual solvents, heavy metals, and product stability.

The improvements in analytical methods has led to improvements in all aspects of botanical medicine preparation, i.e., in harvesting schedules, cultivation techniques, storage, activity, stability of active compounds, and product purity. For example, optimal activity and quality collection should be done at a time when the active ingredient is present in the greatest amount. Improvements in analysis has led to more precise harvesting of many botanicals.

Methods currently utilized in evaluating botanicals and their extracts include organoleptic, microscopic, physical, chemical/physical, and biological. Organoleptic analysis is qualitative and involves the application of sight, odor, taste, touch and occasionally even sound. Microscopic evaluation is indispensable in identifying small fragments of crude or powdered botanicals and in detecting adulterants (e.g., insects, animal feces, mold, fungi, etc.) as well as in identifying the plant by characteristic histological features. Every plant possesses a characteristic histology, which can be demonstrated through study of tissue arrangement, cell walls, and configuration, when properly mounted in stains, reagents, and media.

In crude plant evaluation, physical methods are used to determine solubility, specific gravity, optical rotation, melting point, congealing point, water content, and degree of fiber elasticity. Various chemical/physical methods are also used to determine percentage of active principles, alkaloids, flavonoids, enzymes, vitamins, essential oils, fats, carbohydrates, protein, ash, acid-insoluble ash, or crude fiber present.

The final analytical process requires more precise assays to determine quality, purity, potency, and uniformity. Liquid chromatography, high-pressure liquid chromatography, paper chromatography, thin-layer chromatography, spectrophotometry, atomic absorption, and nuclear magnetic resonance have all been used in the effort to evaluate botanicals and standardize extracts. The plant or extract can then be evaluated by various biological methods, mostly animal tests, to determine pharmacological activity, potency, and toxicity.

Modern herbal preparations

One of the major developments in botanical medicine involves improvements in extraction and concentration processes. An extract is a concentrated form of the herb, obtained by mixing the crude herb with an appropriate solvent and then partially or completely removing the solvent. When an herbal tea bag is steeped in hot water, it is actually a type of herbal extract known as an infusion. The water serves as a solvent in removing some of the medicinal properties from the herb. Teas are often better sources of compounds than the powdered herb but are relatively weak in action compared to tinctures, fluid extracts, and solid extracts.

Herbal tinctures are made using an alcohol and water mixture as the solvent. The herb is soaked in the alcohol solution for a specific amount of time, depending on the herb. This soaking time usually is from several hours to several days. However, some herbs may be soaked for much longer periods of time. The solution is then pressed out, yielding the tincture.

Fluid extracts are more concentrated than tinctures. They are made by distilling off some of the alcohol, typically by using methods that do not require elevated temperatures, such as vacuum distillation and chromatography. Tinctures are often formed by adding alcohol to fluid extracts.

A solid extract is produced by further concentration of the fluid extract, using the mechanisms described. The solvent is completely removed, leaving a viscous extract (soft solid extract) or a dry solid extract, depending on the plant or portion of the plant or on the solvent used. The dry solid extract can be ground into course granules or a fine powder. A solid extract can also be diluted with alcohol and water to form a fluid extract or tincture.

A freeze-dried preparation is produced by freezing the plant material and then exposing it to a very low absolute pressure (high vacuum) and controlled heat input. Under these conditions, the water content is selectively removed via sublimation (i.e., the ice transforms directly to vapor).

Freeze-drying fresh botanicals overcomes two problems often faced when using botanical medicines: lost potency or degradation with time and the undesired use of alcohol. Unfortunately, the process of freeze-drying does not provide a high degree of standardization or concentration of biological activity at this time. Improvements in standardization and concentration of fresh plant materials along with greater pharmacological investigation may make freeze-dried botanicals the preferable form for several plants, particularly those with extremely labile constituents.

In most instances, there is no real comparison between an extract and the ground-dried herb. The extract is more effective, has a higher concentration of active ingredients, has a longer shelf life, and has a greater degree of standardization.

The potencies or strengths of herbal extracts are generally expressed in two ways. If they contain known active principles, their strengths are commonly expressed in terms of the content of these active principles. Otherwise the strength is expressed in terms of their concentration. A 4:1 concentration means that 1 part of the extract is equivalent to, or derived from, 4 parts of the crude herb. This is the typical concentration of a solid extract. One gram of a 4:1 extract is concentrated from 4 g of crude herb.

A tincture is typically a 1:10 or 1:5 concentration, while a fluid extract is usually 1:1. Hence a solid extract is typically at least 4 times as potent when compared to an equal amount of fluid extract and 40 times as potent as a tincture if they are produced from the same quality of herb.

Typically, 1 g of a 4:1 solid extract is equivalent to 4 ml of a fluid extract (⅐ oz) and 40 ml of a tincture (almost 1½ oz).

Quality and the effort to standardize

In the past, the quality of the extract produced was often hard to determine, because many of the active principles of the herbs were unknown. However, recent advances in extraction processes, coupled with improved analytical methods (high-pressure liquid chromatography and thin-layer chromatography) have reduced this problem of quality control. The concentration method of expressing the strength of an extract does not accurately measure potency because there may be great variation between manufacturing techniques and raw materials. By using a high-quality herb (an herb high in active principles), it is possible to have a more potent dried herb, tincture, or fluid extract compared to the solid extract that was made from a lower quality herb. Standardization is the solution to this problem.

If the active components of a particular herb are known (whatever form the herb is in), the herb should be analyzed to ensure that it contains these components at an acceptable standardized level. More accurate dosages can then be given. This form of standardization is generally accepted in Europe and is beginning to be used in the United States as well.

This form of standardization—i.e., stating the content of active constituents versus drug concentration ratio—allows for dosage to be based on active constituents. For example, in Europe, the extract dosage levels of *Vaccinium myrtillus*, *Silybum marianum*, and *Centella asiatica* are based on their active constituent levels rather than on drug ratio or total extract weight. The levels are 40 mg anthocyanosides for *Vaccinium myrtillus*, 70 mg silymarin for *Silybum marianum*, and 30 mg triterpenic acids for *Centella asiatica*. This type of dosage recommendation provides the greatest degree of consistency.

Keep in mind that these extracts are still considered crude extracts and not isolated constituents. For example, an *Uva ursi* extract standardized for its arbutin content (say, 10%) still contains all those synergistic factors that enhance the function of the active ingredient (arbutin).

The future of botanical medicine

As stated earlier, herbs and other plant medicines have been used since antiquity as effective treatments for many common diseases. However, with the advent this century of synthetic drugs, appreciation of plants as medicinal agents has greatly diminished. Currently, there appears to be a renaissance in herbal medicine. It is ironic that this renewal is coming not from traditional herbalists but from renewed scientific investigation into the use of plant medicines. It seems that science and medicine have finally advanced to the point where they can appreciate nature instead of discounting it. The scientific investigation of plant medicines is taking away some of the mystery and romance of herbalism as scientists achieve a greater understanding of the ways in which herbs work. Herbal medicine is being improved by modern scientific research and technology.

Improvements in plant cultivation techniques and the quality of botanical extracts (quality control and standardization) have led to the development of some very effective plant medicines. Many of the "wonder drugs" of the future apparently will be derived from plants or plant cell cultures and from compounds naturally occurring in the human body and produced by cell cultures (interferon, interleukin-II, various hormones, etc.). Several botanical medicines described in this book may in fact already fulfill the role of wonder drug, e.g., *Ginkgo biloba*, *Silybum marianum*, *Panax ginseng*, and *Vaccinium myrtillus*.

The future of botanical medicine in Europe and other parts of the world looks extremely positive. Many of the previous shortcomings of botanical medicine have been overcome (e.g., lack of scientific support, standardization, and quality control). The future of botanical medicine depends on several factors: (1) continued research into botanical medicine, (2) manufacturers' adoption of recognized standards of quality, (3) continued existence of the naturopathic medical schools, and (4) increased public awareness of the tremendous therapeutic value of herbs. Botanical medicine will undoubtedly play a major role in the medicine of the 21st century.

SECTION I

The magic of common food herbs and spices

Too often we forget that the food we eat contains remarkable health-promoting compounds. This first section of this book is dedicated to four common culinary agents: onions, garlic, ginger, and turmeric. Is it possible that these condiments were used initially not only for their ability to enhance the flavor of food but also to preserve food and give it greater medicinal property? I think so.

The herbs discussed in this section serve as examples to highlight the concept that even simple dietary factors can offer significant health benefits. A few years ago I was reading the Sunday newspaper and noticed one of those "ask the doctor" columns. The question featured was, "Does cabbage offer any benefit in the treatment of peptic ulcer?" The doctor's answer was an emphatic *no,* and he went on to elaborate that in his opinion the promotion of folklore is quackery.

His response is most unfortunate for a number of reasons. First, fresh cabbage juice has been well documented in the medical literature as having remarkable success in treating peptic ulcers. In these studies, 1 liter of fresh juice, taken in divided doses, resulted in total ulcer healing in an average of only 10 days. Not only is cabbage juice effective, it is *more* effective than the commonly used prescription drugs the doctor recommended to the inquirer.

I sent a response to the doctor, complete with scientific references, but my letter was never published to my knowledge, nor did I receive a reply.

It is unfortunate that so many people in the medical profession feel threatened that nature may provide solutions. Instead of villifying folklore, we should try to vindicate it. That is exactly what this first section of this book attempts to do with the featured foods—onions, garlic, ginger, and turmeric.

Note: For additional information on therapeutic use of foods, please consult Michael Murray and Joseph Pizzorno, *Encyclopedia of Natural Medicine*, Prima Publishing, Rocklin, CA, 1991.

1

Onion

(ALLIUM CEPA)

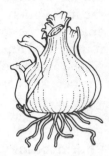

Key uses of onion:

- Infections
- Elevated cholesterol levels
- High blood pressure
- Diabetes
- Asthma

General description

There are numerous forms and varieties of onion, and this perennial or biennial herb is cultivated worldwide. The fleshy bulb is the plant part used. Common varieties are white globe, yellow globe, and red globe.

Chemical composition

Onion, like garlic, contains a variety of organic sulfur compounds, including S-methylcysteine sulfoxide, *trans*-S-(1-propenyl)cysteine sulfoxide, S-propylcysteine sulfoxide, and dipropyl disulfide. Onion also has the enzyme alliinase, which is released when the onion is cut or crushed, causing conversion of *trans*-S-(1-propenyl)cysteine sulfoxide to the so-called lacrimatory (crying) factor (propanethial S-oxide). Other constituents include flavonoids (primarily quercetin), phenolic acids (e.g., caffeic, sinapic, and *p*-coumaric), sterols, saponins, pectin, and volatile oils.[1,2]

History and folk use

Although not as valued a medicinal agent as garlic, onion has been used almost as widely. Like garlic (*Allium sativum*), onion has been used as an antispasmodic, a carminative, a diuretic, an expectorant, a stomachic, an anthelmintic, and an anti-infective agent. (A carminative induces the expulsion of gases; an anthelmintic kills intestinal worms.) Externally it has been used as a rubefacient and a poultice, giving relief in skin diseases and insect bites.[1-3]

Pharmacology

Onion and garlic, because of their similar chemical composition, have many of the same pharmacological effects. There are, however, some significant differences that make one more advantageous than the other in some conditions.

Antimicrobial activity

Although onion does exhibit some antibacterial, antifungal, and anthelmintic activity, it is not nearly as potent as garlic. Although this suggests that garlic may be better indicated in cases of infection,[2-4] onion can usually be consumed in greater quantities than garlic, which may increase the concentration of antimicrobial compounds to approximate those of garlic.

Cardiovascular effects

Like garlic, onions and onion extracts have been shown in several clinical studies to decrease blood lipid levels, prevent clot formation, and lower blood pressure.[5-7] Garlic and onion consumption is associated with lower levels of cholesterol and triglycerides and a lower incidence of atherosclerosis.[8] The quantity of onion consumed during these studies was much greater than that of garlic (600 g of onion per week compared with 50 g of garlic). An argument could be made, therefore, that onion consumption was the major determinant.

Diabetes

Onions have been shown to have significant blood sugar lowering action, comparable to that of the prescription drugs often given to diabetics (tolbutamide and phenformin).[9,10] The active blood sugar lowering principle in onions is believed to be allyl propyl disulphide (APDS), although other constituents, such as flavonoids, may play a significant role as well. Experimental and clinical evidence suggests that APDS lowers glucose by competing with insulin (also a disulfide molecule) for degradation sites in the liver, thereby increasing the life span of insulin. Other mechanisms, such as increased liver metabolism of glucose or increased insulin secretion, have been proposed.

Antiasthmatic action

Onion has been used throughout history as an antiasthmatic agent.[2,3] Onion inhibits the production of compounds that cause the bronchial muscle to spasm. In addition, it relaxes the bronchial muscle.[11,12]

Antitumor effects

An onion extract was found to destroy tumor cells in test tubes and to arrest tumor growth when tumor cells were implanted in rats.[13] The onion extract was shown to be unusually nontoxic; a dose as high as 40 times that of the dose required to kill the tumor cells had no adverse effect on the host. Another species of onion, *Allium ascalonicum* (shallots) has exhibited significant activity against leukemia in mice.[14]

Summary

This discussion on onion highlights its medicinal value, particularly in cardiovascular disease and diabetes mellitus. Because onion is regarded chiefly as a food or seasoning, this raises questions about the medicinal effects of other common vegetables and/or seasonings. Many common vegetables may have significant pharmacological effects that have not yet been investigated. A diet rich in vegetables, spices, or seasonings may offer protection and possibly treatment for a wide variety of diseases. The liberal use of the *Allium* species appears particularly beneficial considering the major disease processes of the 20th century (those processes involved in atherosclerosis, diabetes, and cancer, for example).

Dosage and toxicology

Dosages in the various forms of onion are typically 50–150 g/day (1¾–5 oz/day). There have been virtually no reports of toxicity.

References

1. Leung A: Encyclopedia of Common Natural Ingredients Used in Food, Drugs, and Cosmetics. John Wiley & Sons, New York, NY, 1980. pp246-7
2. Raj KP and Patel NN: Onion - The vegetable drug. Ind Drugs 14:156-60, 1977
3. Vahora SB, Rizwan M, and Khan JA: Medicinal uses of common Indian vegetables. Planta Med 23:381-93, 1973
4. Elnima EI, Ahmed SA, Mekkawi A, and Mossa JS: The antimicrobial activity of garlic and onion extracts. Pharmazie 38:747-8, 1983
5. Louria DB, McAnnally JF, Lasser N, et al: Onion extract in treatment of hypertension and hyperlipidemia: A preliminary communication. Curr Ther Res 37:127-31, 1985
6. Mittal MM, Mittal S, Sarin JC, and Sharma ML: Effects of feeding onion on fibrinolysis, serum cholesterol, platelet aggregation and adhesion. Ind J Med Sci 24:144-8, 1972
7. Menon IS: Fresh onions and blood fibrinolysis. Br Med J i:845, 1969
8. Bever BO and Zahnd GR: Plants with oral hypoglycemic action. Quart J Crude Drug Res 17:139-96, 1979
9. Sharma KK, Gupta RK, Gupta S, and Samuel KC: Antihyperglycemic effect of onion: effect on fasting blood sugar and induced hyperglycemia in man. Ind J Med Res 65:422-9, 1977
10. Dorsch W, Adam O, Weber J, and Ziegeltrum T: Antiasthmatic effects of onion extracts - Detection of benzyl- and other isothiocyanates in mustard oils as antiasthmatic compounds of plant origin. Eur J
11. Pharmacol 107:17-24, 1985
    Dorsch W and Weber J: Prevention of allergen-induced bronchial constriction in sensitized guinea pigs by crude alcohol onion extract. Agents Action 14:626-30, 1984
12. Nepkar DP, Chander R, Bandekar JR, et al: Cytotoxic effect of onion extract on mouse fibrosarcoma 180 A cells. Ind J Exp Biol 19:598-600, 1981
13. Caldes G and Prescott B: A potential antileukemic substance present in Allium ascalonicum. Planta Medica 23:99-100, 1973

2

Garlic

(ALLIUM SATIVUM)

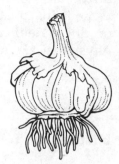

Key uses of garlic:

- Infections
- Elevated cholesterol levels
- High blood pressure
- Diabetes

General description

Garlic, a member of the lily family, is a perennial plant that is cultivated worldwide. The garlic bulb is composed of individual cloves enclosed in a white skin. It is the bulb, either fresh or dehydrated, that is used as a spice or medicinal herb. Garlic oil is obtained by steamed distillation of the crushed fresh bulbs.[1]

Chemical composition

Garlic contains 0.1–0.36% of a volatile oil composed of sulfur-containing compounds: allicin, diallyl disulfide, diallyl trisulfide, and others. These volatile compounds are generally considered to be responsible for most of the pharmacological properties of garlic. Other constituents of garlic include: alliin (S-allyl-L-cysteine sulfoxide), S-methyl-L-cysteine sulfoxide, protein (16.8%, dry weight basis), high concentrations of trace minerals (particularly selenium and germanium), vitamins, glucosinolates, and enzymes (allinase, peroxidase, and myrosinase).[1,2]

Allicin is mainly responsible for the pungent odor of garlic. It is formed by the enzymatic action of alliinase on alliin. The essential oil of garlic yields approximately 60% of its weight in allicin after exposure to alliinase. The enzyme is inactivated by heat, which accounts for the fact that cooked garlic produces neither as strong an odor as raw garlic nor nearly as powerful physiological effects.[21]

History and folk use

Garlic has been used throughout history for the treatment of a wide variety of conditions. Its use predates written history. Sanskrit records document the use of garlic remedies approximately 5,000 years ago, and the Chinese have been using it for at least 3,000 years. The Codex Ebers, an Egyptian medical papyrus dating from about 1550 B.C., mentions garlic as an effective remedy for a variety of ailments, including hypertension, headache, bites, worms, and tumors. Hippocrates, Aristotle, and Pliny cited numerous therapeutic uses for garlic. In general, garlic has been used throughout the world to treat coughs, toothache, earache, dandruff, hypertension, atherosclerosis, hysteria, diarrhea, dysentery, diphtheria, vaginitis, and many other conditions.[1-3]

Stories, verse, and folklore give historical documentation to garlic's power. The folklore of garlic includes its alleged ability to ward off vampires. Sir John Harrington in *The Englishman's Doctor*, written in 1609, summarized garlic's virtues and faults:

> Garlic then have power to save from death
> Bear with it though it maketh unsavory breath,
> And scorn not garlic like some that think
> It only maketh men wink and drink and stink.

In 1721, during a widespread plague in Marseilles, four condemned criminals were recruited to bury the dead. The gravediggers proved to be immune to the disease. Their secret was a concoction that consisted of macerated garlic in wine. This drink became known as *vinaigre des quatre voleurs* (four thieves' vinegar) and is still available in France today.

Garlic's antibiotic activity was noted by Pasteur in 1858. This herb was used by Albert Schweitzer in Africa for the treatment of amebic dysentery. It was also used as an antiseptic in the prevention of gangrene during the two world wars.

Pharmacology

Although garlic has a wide range of well-documented effects, its most important clinical effects are antimicrobial and cardiovascular. This discussion of the pharmacology of garlic focuses therefore on these properties. Because many effects of garlic and onion (*Allium cepa*) are quite similar, readers are encouraged to consult Chapter 1, "Onion," where some of garlic's other effects are described in greater detail.

Antimicrobial activity

Garlic has been shown to have broad-spectrum antimicrobial activity against many genera of bacteria, virus, worms, and fungi, as summarized in several works.[4,35] These findings seem to support the use of garlic throughout history in the treatment of a variety of infectious conditions.

Antibacterial activity

In 1944, Huddleson et al. and Cavallito et al. demonstrated that both garlic juice and allicin inhibited the growth of *Staphylococcus, Streptococcus, Bacillus, Brucella,* and *Vibrio* species at low concentrations.[5,6] In more recent studies that used serial dilution and filter paper disk techniques, fresh garlic and vacuum-dried, powdered garlic preparations were found to be effective antibiotic agents against many bacteria, including *Staphylococcus aureus*, alpha- and beta-hemolytic *Streptococcus, Escherichia coli, Proteus vulgaris, Salmonella enteritidis, Citrobacter* sp., *Klebsiella pneumoniae,* and *Mycobacteria*.[4,7,8] In these studies, the antimicrobial effects of garlic were compared to commonly used antibiotics, including penicillin, streptomycin, chloramphenicol, erythromycin, and tetracyclines. Besides confirming garlic's well-known antibacterial effects, the studies demonstrated efficacy in inhibiting the growth of some bacteria that had become resistant to one or more of the antibiotics.

Antifungal activity

Garlic has demonstrated significant antifungal activity against a wide range of fungi.[4,10-15] From a practical perspective, inhibition of fungi that can infect the skin (*Microsporum, Epidermophyton, Trichophyton*) and *Candida albicans* is most significant. Garlic juice applied topically offers an effective alternative in treating a wide variety of fungal skin diseases.[10] Garlic is especially active against *C. albicans*, being more potent than nystatin, gentian violet, and six other reputed antifungal agents.[4,11-13]

Garlic therapy alone has been used effectively to treat cryptococcal meningitis in a major Chinese hospital.[14] Administering the herb intravenously apparently had the greatest therapeutic value in these patients. While garlic significantly inhibits cryptococcus neoformans,[15] its immune stimulatory effects are thought to be a major factor in its efficacy in this high-mortality disease.

Anthelmintic effects

Garlic extracts also have been shown to have anthelmintic activity against common intestinal parasites, including Ascaris lumbricoides (roundworm) and hookworms.[9,29]

Antiviral effects

Garlic's antiviral effects have been demonstrated in two ways. First, in one study, garlic protected mice from infection by the influenza virus. In other studies, garlic has enhanced the production of antibodies when given with influenza vaccine.[9]

Protection against heart disease

Garlic appears to be an important protective factor against atherosclerosis and heart disease.[16,17] In many animal studies, garlic has reduced elevated cholesterol levels. Human studies have also shown that garlic has a lipid-lowering effect, decreasing total serum cholesterol levels while increasing serum HDL-cholesterol levels.[16,17] HDL-cholesterol is a protective factor against heart disease.

In a 1979 population study, Sainani et al. studied three populations of vegetarians in the Jain community in India who consumed differing amounts of garlic and onions.[30,31] Numerous favorable effects on blood lipids, as shown in Table 1, were observed in the group that consumed the greatest amount of onions and garlic. The study is significant because the subjects had nearly identical diets, except in garlic and onion consumption.

Blood pressure lowering activity

Garlic has demonstrated blood pressure lowering action in both experimental animals and humans.[16-20] Garlic has been shown to decrease the systolic pressure by 20–30 mmHg and the diastolic pressure by 10–20 mmHg in hypertensives.[20] The mode of action of garlic as an antihypertensive appears to be related to its lipid-lowering properties.[19]

Table 1 Effects of garlic and onion consumption on serum lipids under carefully matched diets

Garlic/onion consumption	Cholesterol level	Triglyceride level
Garlic 50 g/week onion 600 g/week	159 mg/dL	52 mg/dL
Garlic 10 g/week onion 200 g/week	172 mg/dL	75 mg/dL
No garlic or onion	208 mg/dL	109 mg/dL

Antitumor effects

Hippocrates prescribed eating garlic as treatment for uterine tumors. According to epidemiological data, there appears to be an inverse relationship between cancer rates and garlic consumption. That is, cancer incidence is lowest where garlic consumption is greatest.[2] Garlic extracts and allicin have displayed antitumor effects and are known to inhibit formation of cancer-causing nitrosamine.[22-24]

Anti-inflammatory effects

Garlic extract has demonstrated significant anti-inflammatory activity in experimental models.[2,9] This is probably a result of the inhibition of pro-inflammatory compounds, caused by garlic.

Diabetes mellitus

Garlic has been used often in the treatment of diabetes mellitus because allicin has been shown to have significant hypoglycemic action. This effect is believed to be the result of increased liver metabolism of glucose, an increased release of insulin, and/or an insulin-sparing effect.[25] Allicin and other sulfhydryl compounds in garlic and onion compete with insulin (also a disulfide protein) for insulin-inactivating sites in the liver. This activity results in an increase in free insulin in the bloodstream. It appears, therefore, that an insulin-sparing mechanism is the major factor in the use of garlic for treating diabetes.

Ear infections

Garlic oil, or the oil in which garlic cloves have been cooked, has been a popular folk remedy for earache.[1,2] Clinical use of a fresh slice of garlic applied directly to the damaged tympanic membrane (eardrum) was satisfactory in repairing eardrum perforation in 18 of 19 cases in one study.[26] This method is particularly indicated in adults with traumatic eardrum perforations, if the garlic is applied within 3 weeks of injury, and provided there is no infection and the perforation is no larger than half of the tympanic membrane. The method is as follows:

1. Prepare a fresh clove of garlic carefully: peel it, but leave the transparent epithelium layer tightly attached.
2. Slice off a very thin piece (about 0.2 mm thick), shaping it just large enough to cover the perforation. Keep the epithelium layer tightly attached to the garlic slice.
3. Insert it into the ear canal and carefully push it against the eardrum so that its cut surface hugs the perforation, with the epithelial layer-covered surface facing the external auditory meatus.
4. Pack the external auditory meatus with an alcohol-moistened cotton ball.

Forceful blowing of the nose should be prohibited, and to prevent infection, water should not be allowed into the ear canal. Replace the garlic slice once or twice a week until healing is complete. Stop treatment if the middle ear becomes inflamed or when the perforation is healed.

This healing effect of garlic on perforated tympanic membranes is thought to be related to allicin's antibiotic activity and to garlic's stimulation of the growth of new tissue.[26]

Other effects

It has been reported that with heavy users of garlic there is no need to inject radio-opaque dyes to visualize the renal tract on x-ray.[27] Garlic possesses diuretic, diaphoretic, emmenagogue, and expectorant action.[1,9] It is also a carminative, an antispasmodic, and a digestant, making it useful in cases of flatulence, nausea, vomiting, colic, and dyspepsia.[9,28]

Summary

The therapeutic uses of garlic are quite extensive. Its use as a food should be encouraged, despite its odor, especially in patients with elevated cholesterol levels, heart disease, hypertension, diabetes, candida infections, asthma, infections (particularly respiratory infections), and gastrointestinal disorders. Garlic juice or slices of garlic can be applied topically in cases of fungal infections, ulcerated wounds, pyoderma, and other skin infections. Garlic can be used as a vaginal suppository, or the juice can be used as a douche, to treat vaginitis, particularly infections due to *Candida albicans*. For the rare individual who has contact dermatitis or who develops negative reactions to garlic, simple discontinuation will quickly alleviate the problems.

Dosage

It is difficult to translate data on extracts, oils, juices, powders, and other proprietary preparations into a uniform equivalent. The typical dosage from the positive studies is in the range of 10–30 g (⅓–1 oz) of fresh garlic (about three–eight cloves) per 60 kg of body weight per day.[16] Because many of the therapeutic compounds in garlic have not been found in cooked, processed, and proprietary forms, the broad range of beneficial effects attributed to garlic are best obtained from fresh, raw garlic, although limited, specific effects can be obtained from the other forms.[3] The few negative studies concerning garlic and its cardiovascular effects are hardly worth mentioning because the dosages used in these were only 10–30% of those used in the positive studies.[16,17]

Toxicology

For the vast majority of individuals, garlic is nontoxic at the dosages commonly used. For some people, however, it causes allergic contact dermatitis (eczema)[1,32,33] and irritation to the digestive tract.[17] Others apparently are unable to effectively detoxify allicin and other sulfur-containing components. Prolonged consumption of large amounts of raw garlic by rats resulted in anemia, weight loss, and failure to grow.[34]

References

1. Leung A: Encyclopedia of Common Natural Ingredients Used in Food, Drugs, and Cosmetics. John Wiley & Sons, New York, NY, 1980. pp176-8
2. Raj KP and Parmar RM: Garlic - condiment and medicine. Ind Drugs 15:205-10, 1977
3. Block E: The chemistry of garlic and onions. Scientific American, March 1985. pp114-8
4. Adetumbi MA and Lau BH: Allium sativum (garlic) - A natural antibiotic. Med Hypothesis 12:227-37, 1983
5. Huddleson IF, DuFrain J, Barrons KC, and Giefel M: Antibacterial substances in plants. J Am Vet Med Assoc 105:394-7, 1944
6. Cavallito CJ and Bailey JH: Allicin, the antibacterial principle of allium sativum. I. Isolation, physical properties and antibacterial action. J Am Chem Soc 66:1950-1, 1944
7. Sharma VD, Sethi MS, Kumar PS, and Rarotra JR: Antibacterial property of Allium sativum Linn.: in vivo & in vitro studies. Ind J Exp Biol 15:466-8, 1977
8. Elnima EI, Ahmed SA, Mekkawi A, and Mossa JS: The antimicrobial activity of garlic and onion extracts. Pharmazie 38:747-8, 1983

9. Vahora SB, Rizwan M, and Khan JA: Medicinal uses of common Indian vegetables. Planta Med 23:381-93, 1973
10. Amer M, Taha M, and Tosson Z: The effect of aqueous garlic extract on the growth of dermatophytes. Int J Dermatol 19:285-7, 1980
11. Moore GS and Atkins RD: The fungicidal and fungistatic effects of an aqueous garlic extract on medically important yeast-like fungi. Mycologia 69:341-8, 1977
12. Sandhu DK, Warraich MK and Singh S: Sensitivity of yeasts isolated from cases of vaginitis to aqueous extracts of garlic. Mykosen 23:691-8, 1980
13. Prasad G and Sharma VD: Efficacy of garlic (Allium sativum) treatment against experimental candidiasis in chicks. Br Vet J 136:448-51, 1980
14. Garlic in cryptococcal meningitis. A preliminary report of 21 cases. Chinese Med J 93:123-6, 1980
15. Fromtling R and Bulmer G: In vitro effect of aqueous extract of garlic (Allium sativum) on the growth and viability of cryptococcus neoformans. Mycologia 70:397-405, 1978
16. Norwell DY and Tarr RS: Garlic, vampires, and CHD. Osteopathic Annals 11:546-9, 1983
17. Lau BH, Adetumbi MA, and Sanchez A: Allium sativum (garlic) and atherosclerosis: A review. Nutri Research 3:119-28, 1983
18. Malik ZA and Siddiqui S: Hypotensive effect of freeze-dried garlic (Allium sativum) sap in dog. J Pakistan Med Assoc 31:12-3, 1981
19. Petkov V: Plants with hypotensive, antiatheromatous and coronary dilating action. Am J Chin Med 7:197-236, 1979
20. Foushee DB, Ruffin J, and Banerjee U: Garlic as a natural agent for the treatment of hypertension: A preliminary report. Cytobios 34:145-62, 1982
21. Chutani SK and Bordia A: The effect of fried versus raw garlic on fibrinolytic activity in man. Atherosclerosis 38:417-21, 1981
22. Choy YM, Kwok TT, Fung KP, and Lee CY: Effect of garlic, Chinese Medicinal drugs and amino acids on growth of Erlich ascites tumor cells in mice. Am J Chinese Med 11:69-73, 1982
23. Weisberger AS and Pensky J: Tumor inhibition by a sulfhydryl-blocking agent related to an active principle of garlic (Allium sativum). Cancer Research 18:1301-8, 1958
24. Xing M, Wang ML, Xu HX, et al: Garlic and gastric cancer - the effect of garlic on nitrite and nitrate in gastric juice. Acta Nutri Sinica 4:53-5, 1982
25. Bever BO and Zahnd GR: Plants with oral hypoglycemic action. Quart J Crude Drug Res 17:139-96, 1979
26. Wei-cheng H: Garlic slice in repairing eardrum perforation. Chinese Med J 3:204-5, 1977
27. Macpherson RL: Garlic pyelography. Lancet ii:732, 1973
28. Barowsky H and Boyd LJ: The use of garlic (Allistan) in gastrointestinal disturbances. Rev Gastroenterol 11:22-6, 1944
29. Bastidas GJ: Effect of ingested garlic on Necator americanus and Ancylostoma canium. Am J Trop Med Hyg 18:920-3, 1969
30. Sainani GS, Desai DB, Gorhe NH, et al: Effect of dietary garlic and onion on serum lipid profile in the Jain community. Ind J Med Res 69:776-80, 1979
31. Sainani GS, Desai DB, Gorhe NH, et al: Dietary garlic, onion and some coagulation parameters in Jain community. J Assoc Phys Ind 27:707-12, 1979
32. Bleumink E, Doeglas HMG, Klokke AH and Nater JP: Allergic contact dermatitis to garlic. Br J Dermatol 87:6-9, 1972
33. Vanketal WG and Dehaan P: Occupational eczema from garlic and onion. Contact Dermatitis 4:53-64, 1978
34. Nakagawa S, Masamoto K, Sumiyoshi H, et al: Effect of raw and extracted-aged garlic juice on growth of young rats and their organs after perioral administration. J Toxicol Sci 5:91-112, 1980
35. Reichenberg J: A scientific basis for the active principle of garlic (Allium sativum) and its use as a hypocholesterolemic and antibacterial/antifungal agent. J John Bastyr Col Nat Med 2:28-32, 1980

3

Ginger

(ZINGIBER OFFICINALE)

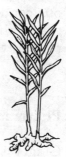

Key uses of ginger:

- Nausea and vomiting of pregnancy
- Motion sickness
- Vertigo
- Arthritis

General description

Ginger is an upright perennial herb with thick tuberous rhizomes (underground stems and root) from which the aerial stem grows up to 1 m in height. It is native to southern Asia, although it is extensively cultivated in the tropics (e.g., India, China, Jamaica, Haiti, and Nigeria). Exports from Jamaica to all parts of the world amount to more than 2 million pounds annually. Extracts and dried ginger are produced from dried unpeeled ginger because peeled ginger loses much of its essential oil content.[1,2]

Chemical composition

The following compounds have been isolated from ginger: starch (up to 50%); protein (about 9%); lipids (6–8%), composed of triglycerides, phosphatidic acid, lecithins, free fatty acids; a protease, or protein-digesting enzyme (2.26%); volatile oils (1–3%), the principle components of which are three sesquiterpenes (bisabolene, zingiberene, and zingiberol); vitamins (especially niacin and vitamin A); and resins.[1,2]

History and folk use

Dried ginger has been used for thousands of years in China to treat numerous conditions, including stomachache, diarrhea, nausea, cholera, hemorrhage, rheumatism, and toothache.[1] In the United States, ginger has been primarily used as a carminative, diaphoretic, appetite stimulant, and local irritant.[3]

Pharmacology

Ginger is reported to have numerous pharmacological properties, including anti-inflammatory action, positive effects on the liver, cholesterol-lowering effects, heart tonifying action, many beneficial effects on the gastrointestinal tract, and an ability to relieve motion sickness and dizziness.[1-12]

Anti-inflammatory action

The aqueous (water) extract of ginger has been shown to be a very potent inhibitor of the formation of inflammatory compounds (prostaglandin and thromboxanes).[5] This effect may help to explain the use of ginger throughout history as an anti-inflammatory agent. However, ginger and its extracts also have strong antioxidant activities and contain a protease that may have similar action to other plant proteases (e.g., bromelain, ficin, and papain) on inflammation.[1]

In one clinical study, seven patients with rheumatoid arthritis, for whom conventional drugs had provided only temporary or partial relief, were treated with ginger. One patient took 50 g/day of lightly cooked ginger; the remaining six patients took either 5 g of fresh ginger or 0.1–1 g of powdered ginger daily. All patients reported substantial improvement, including pain relief, joint mobility, and decrease in swelling and morning stiffness.[12]

Liver, cholesterol, and bile effects

Ginger has been shown to significantly reduce serum and liver cholesterol levels in cholesterol-fed rats by impairing cholesterol absorption and improving liver function.[6] The ability of ginger to lower cholesterol levels within the liver is largely a result of its choleretic effect.[9] Choleretics are substances that promote the flow of bile from the liver to the gallbladder and small intestine. Cholesterol is converted to bile within the liver; presumably this is stimulated by ginger. Often, cholesterol cannot be converted to bile acids, which results in an increased risk for gallstones and damage to the liver.

Bile is necessary for the absorption of fats, fat-soluble vitamins, and various other compounds. Perhaps many of ginger's digestion-improving effects are a result of this herb stimulating bile secretion.

Gastrointestinal and antivertigo effects

Historically, the majority of complaints for which ginger was used concerned the gastrointestinal system. It is generally regarded as an excellent carminative (a substance that promotes the elimination of intestinal gas) and an intestinal spasmolytic (a substance that relaxes and soothes the intestinal tract).

A clue to ginger's efficacy in eliminating gastrointestinal distress is offered by recent double-blind studies, which demonstrated that ginger is very effective in preventing the symptoms of motion sickness, especially seasickness.[8,10,11] In fact, in one study, ginger was shown to be far superior to Dramamine, a commonly used over-the-counter and prescription drug for motion sickness. Ginger reduces all symptoms associated with motion sickness, including dizziness, nausea, vomiting, and cold sweating.[8,10,11]

Ginger has long been used in the treatment of nausea and vomiting associated with pregnancy. Recently, the efficacy of ginger was confirmed in the most severe form of nausea and vomiting during pregnancy (*hyperemesis gravidarum*). This condition usually requires hospitalization. Ginger root powder at a dose of 250 mg four times a day brought about a significant reduction in both the severity of the nausea and the number of attacks of vomiting.[13]

Summary

Ginger is more than a condiment; it is a valuable therapeutic agent. Its safety and effectiveness are particularly evident in morning sickness of pregnancy, nausea, and motion sickness.

Dosage

In general, ginger, like many other herbs and spices, can be used liberally. The dose used in the treatment of motion sickness, vertigo, and nausea and vomiting during pregnancy is 1 g of powdered ginger root.

Toxicology

There does not appear to be any toxicity associated with ginger root ingestion.

References

1. Leung A: Encyclopedia of Common Natural Ingredients Used in Food, Drugs, and Cosmetics. John Wiley & Sons, New York, NY, 1980. pp184-6
2. Tyler V, Brady L and Robbers J: Pharmacognosy. 8th ed, Lea & Febiger, Philadelphia, PA 1981. pp156-7
3. Felter H: The Eclectic Materia Medica, Pharmacology and Therapeutics. Eclectic Medical Publications, Portland, Or, 1983. p702
4. Srivastava K: Effects of aqueous extracts of onion, garlic and ginger on the platelet aggregation and metabolism of arachidonic acid in the blood vascular system: In vitro study. Prost Leukotri Med 13:227-35, 1984
5. Kiuchi F, Shibuyu M and Sankawa U: Inhibitors of prostaglan din biosynthesis from ginger. Chem Pharm Bull 30:754-7, 1982
6. Gujral S, Bhumra H and Swaroop M: Effect of ginger (Zingebar officinate Roscoe) oleoresin on serum and hepatic cholesterol levels in cholesterol fed rats. Nutr Rep Intl 17:183-9, 1978
7. Shoji N, Iwasa A, Takemoto T, Ishida Y and Ohizumi Y: Cardiotonic principles of ginger (Zingiber officinale Roscoe). J Pharm Sci 10:1174-5, 1982
8. Mowrey D and Clayson D: Motion sickness, ginger, and psychophysics. Lancet i:655-7, 1982
9. Yamahara J, Miki K, Chisaka T, et al: Cholagogic effect of ginger and its active constituents. J Ethnopharmacol. 13:217-25, 1985
10. Grontved A and Hentzer E: Vertigo-reducing effect of ginger root. ORL 48:282-6, 1986
11. Grontved A, Brask T, Kambskard J and Hentzer E: Ginger root against seasickness. A controlled trial on the open sea. Acta Otolaryngol 105:45-9, 1988
12. Srivastava KC and Mustafa T: Ginger (Zingiber officinale) and rheumatic disorders. Med Hypothesis 29:25-28, 1989
13. Fischer-Rasmussen W, Kjaer SK, Dahl C and Asping U: Finger treatment of hyperemesis gravidarum. Eur J Ob Gyn Reproductive Biol 38:19-24, 1990

4

Turmeric

(CURCUMA LONGA)

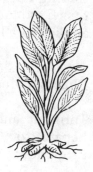

Key uses of turmeric and curcumin (a component of the plant):

- Inflammation
- Arthritis
- Gallbladder infection or inflammation
- Liver disorders

General description

Curcuma longa is a perennial herb of the ginger family. It is cultivated extensively in India, China, Indonesia, and other tropical countries. It has a thick rhizome from which arise large, oblong, and long-petioled leaves. The rhizome (root) is the part used; it is usually cured (boiled, cleaned, and sundried) and polished.[1]

Chemical composition

Turmeric contains 4–5% of an orange-yellow volatile oil that is composed mainly of turmerone, atlantone, and zingiberone; 0.3–5.4% curcumin; sugars (28% glucose, 12% fructose, 1% arabinose); resins; protein; some vitamins; and some minerals.[1]

History and folk use

Turmeric is the major ingredient in curry powder. It is also used in prepared mustard. It is extensively used both for its color and flavor.

Turmeric is used in both the Chinese and Indian systems of medicine as an anti-inflammatory agent and in the treatment of numerous conditions, including flatulence, jaundice, menstrual difficulties, bloody urine, hemorrhage, toothache, bruises, chest pain, and colic.[1] Turmeric poultices are often applied locally to relieve inflammation and pain.

Pharmacology

Turmeric and its derivatives have exhibited anti-inflammatory and anti-hepatotoxic (liver-protecting) effects.[1,2] The pharmacology and potency of turmeric are believed to be caused by its volatile oil and curcumin content.

Anti-inflammatory effects

The volatile oil fraction of C. *longa* has been demonstrated to possess significant anti-inflammatory activity in a variety of experimental models.[3,4] Even more potent in acute inflammation is the yellow pigment of turmeric, curcumin (diferuloyl methane).[5-7] Curcumin and curcumin analogs are believed to be the main pharmacological agents in turmeric. Curcumin's effects in these studies were comparable to the potent drugs hydrocortisone and phenylbutazone. While these drugs are associated with significant toxicity (e.g., ulcer formation, and decreased white blood cell numbers), turmeric displays no toxicity.

Although a number of hypotheses have been formulated, no clear-cut mechanism for curcumin's anti-inflammatory action has been determined.[5,6] It is known that curcumin is much less active in animals that have had their adrenal glands removed, which suggests an indirect action through the adrenal cortex. This, however, is inconsistent with findings that show it does not stimulate release of steroids like cortisone by the adrenal cortex or produce any significant change in the adrenal ascorbic acid and cholesterol levels (which should be lowered if adrenal activity is increased).[5,6] Other possible explanations are that curcumin sensitizes or primes cortisone receptor sites, thereby potentiating cortisone action, or that curcumin increases the life span of cortisone in the body by inhibiting cortisone breakdown in the liver.

Curcumin also has some significant direct effects, including inhibiting leukotriene formation, inhibiting platelet aggregation, promoting the breakdown of fibrin, inhibiting neutrophil response to various stimuli involved in the inflammatory process, stabilizing lysosomal membranes, and a number of beneficial effects on liver function.[5,6,10,11]

Clinical studies have substantiated curcumin's anti-inflammatory effects, including a clinical effect in rheumatoid arthritis.[12,13] In this study, curcumin was compared to phenylbutazone. The improvements in the duration of morning stiffness, walking speed, and joint swelling were comparable in both groups.[12] In a new human model for evaluating NSAIDs (postoperative inflammation model), 400 mg of curcumin was comparable to 100 mg of phenylbutazone.[13]

It must be pointed out that while curcumin has an anti-inflammatory effect similar to phenylbutazone and various NSAIDs, it does not possess as potent direct analgesic action. Although 60% of orally administered curcumin is absorbed,[14,15] absorption may be improved when curcumin is administered with bromelain or other proteolytic enzymes.

Liver effects

The components of turmeric prevent the liver from being damaged by toxic chemicals and enhances the flow of bile (a choleretic effect).[5,8] These results support turmeric's historical use in treating liver disorders. In addition, alcohol extracts and the essential oil of C. longa have been shown to inhibit the growth of most organisms that can cause inflammation of the gallbladder.

Summary

Curcumin may be the most potent anti-inflammatory compound in botanical medicine. The action of curcumin is comparable to potent drugs, yet curcumin's toxicity is substantially less than with potent drugs. C. longa and curcumin also have a beneficial effect in preventing liver damage and promoting the flow of bile.

Dosage

Obviously, turmeric can be consumed liberally in the diet. For medicinal effects, curcumin is recommended at a dose of 250–500 mg three times a day. The use of bromelain in conjunction with curcumin may provide the greatest advantage due to bromelain's anti-inflammatory action and its ability to possibly enhance the absorption of curcumin.

Toxicology

Toxicity reactions to turmeric or curcumin have not been reported. Extremely high doses of turmeric, its alcohol extracts, and curcumin have not produced any side effects in either mice, rats, guinea pigs, or monkeys.[5,7,9]

References

1. Leung A: Encyclopedia of Common Natural Ingredients Used in Food, Drugs, and Cosmetics. John Wiley & Sons, New York, NY, 1980 pp313-4
2. Lutomski VJ, Kedzia B and Debska W: Effect of an alcohol extract and active ingredients from Curcuma longa on bacteria and fungi. Planta Med 26:17-9 ,1974
3. Chandra D and Gupta S: Anti-inflammatory and anti-arthritic activity of volatile oil of curcuma longa (Haldi). Ind J Med Res 60:138-42, 1972
4. Arora R, Basu N, Kapoor V and Jain A: Anti-inflammatory studies on curcuma longa (turmeric). Ind J Med Res 59:1289-95, 1971
5. Srimal R and Dhawan B: Pharmacology of diferuloyl methane (curcumin), a non-steroidal anti-inflammatory agent. J Pharm Pharmac 25:447-52, 1973
6. Mukhopadhyay A, Basu N, Ghatak N and Gujral P: Anti-inflammatory and irritant activities of curcumin analogues in rats. Agents Actions 12:508-15, 1982
7. Ghatak N and Basu N: Sodium curcuminate as an effective anti-inflammatory agent. Ind J Exp Biol 10:235-6, 1972
8. Kiso Y, Suzuki Y, Watanabe N, et al: Antihepatotoxic principles of curcuma longa rhizomes. Planta Med 49:185-7, 1983
9. Shankar TNB, Shantha NV, Ramesh HP, et al: Toxicity studies on turmeric (Curcuma longa): Acute toxicity studies in rats, guinea pigs & monkeys. Indian J Exp Biol 18:73-5,1980
10. Srivastava R and Srimal RC: Modification of certain inflammation-induced biochemical changes by curcumin. Indian J Med Res 81:215-23, 1985
11. Srivastava R: Inhibition of neutrophil response by curcumin. Agents Actions 28:298-303, 1989
12. Deodhar SD, Sethi R and Srimal RC: Preliminary studies on antirheumatic activity of curcumin (diferuloyl methane). Ind J Med Res 71:632-4, 1980
13. Satoskar RR, Shah SJ and Shenoy SG: Evaluation of anti-inflammatory property of curcumin (diferuloyl methane) in patients with postoperative inflammation. Int J Clin Pharmacol Ther Toxicol 24:651-4, 1986
14. Wahlstrom B and Blennow G: A study on the fate of curcumin in the rat. Acta Pharmacol Toxicol 43:86-92, 1978
15. Ravindranath V and Chandrasekhara N: Absorption and tissue distribution of curcumin in rats. Toxicology 16:259-65, 1980

SECTION II

Herbal tonics

Herbs that work on the body as a whole, heightening the general tone by improving the processes of the circulatory, hormonal, nervous, and digestive systems, are known as tonics. Many herbs fulfill this general definition of a tonic; many others are specific system tonics, e.g., uterine tonic, digestive tonic, and liver tonic.

In this section, three of the more popular tonics are discussed: Chinese ginseng, Siberian ginseng, and dong quai (often referred to as the "female's ginseng"). Although women can gain as much benefit from ginseng as men, for some reason the use of ginseng in the United States has been much more popular with men than women.

It has been said that the use of herbal tonics is like giving an engine a tune-up; the use of herbal stimulants (like coffee and tea) is like stepping on the gas pedal. What should be most apparent from reading the descriptions of these herbs are the tremendous abilities of the herbs in restoring balance in the body.

5

Chinese or Korean ginseng

(PANAX GINSENG)

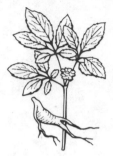

Key uses of Panax ginseng:

- Recovery from illness
- Stress
- Performance enhancement
- Diabetes
- Enhancement of sexual function
- Protection against radiation

General description

Korean or Chinese ginseng is a small perennial plant that originally grew wild in the damp woodlands of northern China, Manchuria, and Korea. Wild ginseng is now extremely rare. However, ginseng is a widely cultivated plant, especially in Korea, but also in Russia, China, and Japan. In addition to *Panax ginseng* C. A. Meyer, four other closely related species are often used: *P. quinquefolium* (American ginseng), *P. japonicum* C. A. Meyer (Japanese ginseng), *P. pseudoginseng* (Himalayan ginseng), and *P. trifolium. P. ginseng* C. A. Meyer is the most widely used and most extensively studied species. Its pharmacology is the major focus of this chapter.[1,2]

Fully mature, Korean ginseng is a herbaceous plant with a taproot, five-lobed palmate leaves, and greenish-white flowers in an umbel. The first year, ginseng bears only a single leaf with three leaflets. In the second year, it bears a single leaf with five leaflets, and in its third year, it bears two leaves with five leaflets. It usually starts flowering in its fourth year, while bearing three leaves. The roots of the cultivated plant are 3–4 mm in diameter and 10 cm long, whereas the roots of wild plants may attain 10 cm in diameter and a length of 50–60 cm.

Ginseng is often processed in two forms: white and red ginseng. White ginseng is the dried root, and its peripheral skin is frequently peeled off. Red ginseng is the steamed root, which shows a caramel-like color.[2]

There are many types and grades of ginseng and ginseng extracts, depending on the source, age, and parts of the root used and on the methods of preparation. Old, wild, well-formed roots are the most valued, and rootlets of cultivated plants are considered the lowest grade. For largely economic purposes, the majority of ginseng in the American marketplace has been derived from the lowest grade of root, diluted with excipients, blended with adulterants, or it is totally devoid of active constituents, that is, ginsenosides.[3]

High-quality roots and extracts are available, however. These preparations are the main root of plants between 4 and 6 years of age, or of extracts that have been standardized for ginsenoside content and ratio to ensure optimum pharmacological effect.

Chemical composition

Ginseng contains at least 13 different triterpenoid saponins, collectively known as ginsenosides, which are believed to be the most important active constituents. The usual concentration of ginsenosides is between 1 and 3%. The ginsenosides have been designated R_0, R_{b1}, R_{b2}, R_{b3}, R_c, R_d, R_e, R_f, 20-gluco-R_f, R_{g1}, and R_{g2}. The ginsenosides differ primarily in the sugar groups that are attached to the steroid molecule.

Ginsenosides R_{b1}, R_{b2}, R_c, R_e, and R_{g1} are present in significant concentrations in Korean ginseng. In contrast, American ginseng (*Panax quinquefolium*) contains primarily ginsenosides R_{b1} and R_e, and does not contain ginsenosides R_{b2}, R_f, or, in some instances, R_{g1}. This allows for easy detection of species using HPLC (high-pressure liquid chromatography).[1,2,4]

Other components include panacene, a volatile oil; free and glucoside-bound sterols (e.g., beta-sitosterol and its beta-glucoside); polyacetylene derivatives B-elemene and panaxinol; 8–32% starch; low molecular weight polysaccharides; pectin; vitamins (e.g., thiamin, riboflavin, B_{12}, nicotinic acid, pantothenic acid, and biotin); 0.1–0.2% choline; minerals; simple sugars (glucose, fructose, sucrose, maltose, trisaccharides, etc.); and various flavonoids.[1,2,4]

Although it had been reported that ginseng contains large amounts of germanium (i.e., 300 ppm), a follow-up study using highly sensitive (detection limit of 1 ppb), flameless atomic absorption spectrometry combined with solvent extraction demonstrated that the highest concentration of germanium measured in samples of ginseng purchased in the Osaka market was only 6 ppb.[65] More research is needed to accurately determine the germanium content of botanical medicines, because the reported concentrations vary widely. Such low levels suggest that a connection between the pharmacology of ginseng and its germanium content is unlikely.

History and folk use

Perhaps the most famous medicinal plant of China, ginseng generally has been used alone or in combination with other herbs to restore the "yang" quality. It has also been used as a tonic for its revitalizing properties, especially after long illnesses. Ginseng is used in folk medicine for amnesia, anemia, anorexia, asthma, atherosclerosis, boils, bruises, cachexia, cancer, convulsions, cough, debility, diabetes, divination, dysentery, dysmenorrhea, dyspepsia, enterorrhagia, epilepsy, epistaxis, fatigue, fear, fever, forgetfulness, gastritis, hangover, headache, heart, hematoptysis, hemorrhage, hyperglycemia, hypertension, hypotension, impotence, insomnia, intestinal complaints, longevity promotion, malaria, menorrhagia, nausea, neurasthenia, palpitations, polyuria, pregnancy, puerperium, rectocele, rhinitis, rheumatism, shortness of breath, sores, spermatorrhea, splenitis, swelling, and vertigo. It has been used as an alterative, anodyne, aperitif, aphrodisiac, cardiotonic, carminative, diuretic, emetic, estrogenic, expectorant, gonadotrophic, nervine, sedative, sialogogue, stimulant, stomachic, and tranquilizer.[1,5]

As can be seen from this list, ginseng has been used for most conditions, reflecting a broad range of nutritional and medicinal properties.

Pharmacology

Since the 1950s, a great amount of research has been conducted worldwide to determine whether the therapeutic properties attributed to ginseng belong in the realm of legend or fact. Unfortunately, inconsistent results (mostly from different procedures in the preparation of extracts, the use of nonofficial parts of the plant, the use of adulterants, and the lack of quality control in the ginseng used) have made determination of ginseng's true properties difficult. Nonetheless, enough good research does exist to indicate that ginseng possesses pharmacological activity consistent with its near-legendary status, especially when high-quality extracts, standardized for active constituents, are used.

Over the years, ginseng has been reported to have numerous pharmacological effects in humans and laboratory animals, including general

40

stimulatory effects during stress; decrease in sensitivity to stress; increase in mental and physical capacity for work; improved endocrine system function; resistance to radiation sickness, experimental neurosis, and cancer; enhanced protein synthesis and cell reproduction; improved glucose control in humans and alloxan-induced diabetes in rats; modulation of various immune system parameters; lowering of serum cholesterol; and protection of the liver from toxic substances.[1,2,4,5] Some of these actions are discussed in greater detail below.

Adaptogenic activity

Ginseng was originally investigated for its adaptogen qualities. An adaptogen was defined in 1957 by the Russian pharmacologist I. I. Brekhman as a substance that (1) must be innocuous and cause minimal disorders in the physiological functions of an organism, (2) must have a nonspecific action (i.e., it should increase resistance to adverse influences by a wide range of physical, chemical, and biochemical factors), and (3) usually has a normalizing action irrespective of the direction of the pathologic state.[2] According to tradition and scientific evidence, ginseng possesses this kind of equilibrating, tonic, antistress action, and so the term *adaptogen* is quite appropriate in describing its general effects.[2,6,7]

From a practical perspective, ginseng can be used as a general tonic, especially in debilitated and feeble individuals. Use in this manner is consistent with its historic application.

Antifatigue (mental and physical) activity

Some of the first studies of ginseng's adaptogenic activities were performed during the late 1950s and early 1960s by Brekhman and Dardymov in the U.S.S.R. and by Petkov in Bulgaria.[6-10]

In one of Brekhman's experiments, Soviet soldiers given an extract of ginseng ran faster in a 3-km race than those given a placebo. In another experiment, radio operators tested after administration of ginseng extract transmitted text significantly faster and with fewer mistakes than those given a placebo. These and similar results found by European researchers, who demonstrated improvement in human physical and mental performance after the administration of ginseng extracts, prompted researchers to confirm the results in experimental models using mice.[2,6-8]

In perhaps the best known of these experiments, mice were subjected to swimming in cold water or running up an apparently endless rope to determine if ginseng could increase the time to exhaustion. The results indicated that ginseng possessed significant antifatigue activity because the experimenters noted a clear dose-dependent increase in time to exhaustion in mice receiving ginseng.[2,7,11-14] In one study, the time to exhaustion was increased up to 183% in the mice given ginseng 30 min prior to exercising, compared with controls.[7]

Experimental animal studies indicated that much of the antifatigue action of ginseng was due to the stimulant effect of ginseng on the central nervous system (the brain and spinal cord, abbreviated CNS). Ginseng ingestion improves energy metabolism during prolonged exercise.[9-14]

Ginseng has been shown to increase muscle stimulation by nerve impulses,[15] modify brain-wave tracings,[9] improve metabolic activity in the brain,[16] and affect the hypothalamo-pituitary-adrenal axis, all of which could be largely responsible for ginseng's antifatigue activity on mental and physical performance. The CNS activity of ginseng is essentially different from that of the usual stimulants. Although stimulants are active under most situations, ginseng reveals its stimulatory action only under the challenge of stress.[16]

On the physical level, ginseng's antifatigue properties appear closely related to its ability to spare glycogen utilization in exercising muscle.[13] Glycogen is the storage form of glucose (a sugar) in muscle. Exercise physiologists have clearly established that during prolonged exercise, the development of fatigue is closely related to the depletion of glycogen stores and the build-up of lactic acid, both in skeletal muscle and the liver. If an adequate supply of oxygen is available to the working muscle, fatty acids are the preferred source for energy production, thus sparing utilization of muscle glycogen. The greater the ability to conserve body glycogen stores by using fatty acids as the energy source, the greater the amount of time to exhaustion. Ginseng enhances the breakdown of fatty acids to energy during prolonged exercise, thereby sparing muscle glycogen stores.[13]

The mental and physical antifatigue effects of ginseng have been demonstrated in both animal studies and double-blind, clinical trials in humans. In addition to several Russian studies using soldiers and athletes as subjects, other studies have been published.[17,18]

In one double-blind, clinical study, nurses who had switched from day to night duty rated themselves for competence, mood, and general well-being and were given a test for mental and physical performance along with blood cell counts and blood chemistry evaluation. The group taking ginseng demonstrated higher scores in competence, mood parameters, and mental and physical performance when compared with those receiving a placebo.[17]

In a double-blind, cross-over study on university students in Italy, ginseng extract was compared with a placebo in various tests of mental performance. A favorable effect of ginseng relative to baseline performance was observed in attention, mental arithmetic, logical deduction, integrated brain-body function, and reaction time to sounds. It is interesting to note that in the course of the trial, the students taking ginseng reported a greater sensation of well-being.[18]

From a practical standpoint, ginseng's antifatigue properties may be useful whenever fatigue or lack of energy is apparent. Athletes, in particular, may derive some benefit from ginseng use.

Antistress activity

Stress is a term widely used in our current fast-paced society. Often the demands placed on us daily build and accumulate to a point where we find it almost impossible to cope. Job pressures, family arguments, financial pressures, and deadlines on the job are all common examples of stressors. Actually, a stressor may be almost anything that creates a disturbance, including exposure to heat or cold, environmental toxins, toxins produced by microorganisms, physical trauma, and, of course, strong emotional reactions to various stimuli.

Ginseng has been shown to enhance the ability to cope with various stressors, both physical and mental. Presumably this is a result of delaying the alarm phase (fight or flight) response in Selye's classic model of stress. Much of ginseng's antistress effects are due to its effect on the adrenal glands,[4,13,19,20] which are responsible for maintaining the balance of many bodily functions during stress by secreting several important hormones.

Italian researchers have studied the effect of a standardized ginseng extract on rats exposed to cold.[4,19] The ginseng extract significantly counteracted body temperature decline without affecting blood glucose or cortisone levels. In a group of rats that had their adrenal glands surgically removed, the ginseng extract had no significant effects. This study demonstrated that ginseng's antistress effect was dependent on adrenal function.

It appears, based on extensive research, that ginseng acts through nervous system control mechanisms to adjust metabolic and functional systems that maintain the body during the challenge of stresses.[11,12] This is very similar to how a thermostat maintains temperature.

Researchers have demonstrated that ginseng acts predominantly on the hypothalamus and pituitary to promote secretion of adrenocorticotropic hormone (ACTH), a hormone that promotes the manufacture and secretion of adrenal hormones.[21,22] This release of ACTH and associated pituitary substances (e.g., beta-lipoprotein, endorphins, enkephalins, etc.), is probably responsible for many of the antifatigue and antistress actions of ginseng because ACTH and adrenal hormones have been shown to bind directly to brain tissue to increase mental activities during stress.

From a practical perspective, it is apparent that ginseng has a balancing effect on the hypothalamic-pituitary-adrenal axis by adjusting metabolic and functional systems governing hormonal control of homeostasis.[20-22] This assists the body's response to the challenge of stress and therefore is indicated when disruption of this axis is apparent.

Ginseng may prove especially effective in restoring normal adrenal function and preventing adrenal atrophy associated with corticosteroid administration. In rats, ginseng has been found to inhibit cortisone-induced adrenal and thymic atrophy.[23]

Several other herbs also possess adrenal-enhancing activity, most notably Chinese thoroughway (*Bupleuri falcatum*)[24], licorice (*Glycyrrhiza glabra*),[25] turmeric (*Curcuma longa*),[26] and Siberian ginseng (*Eleutherococcus senticosus*).[27]

Effects with diabetes

Ginseng, used either alone or in combination with other botanicals, has a long folk use in the treatment of diabetes. Ginseng has confirmed hypoglycemic or blood sugar lowering activity. The ginseng components responsible for this effect include five types of substances: five glycans (polysaccharides designated panaxans A to E), adenosine, a carboxylic acid, a peptide, and a fraction designated DPG-3-2.[28-32] The ginsenosides are devoid of hypoglycemic action, a fact that highlights the importance of using crude, standardized extracts containing all active principles versus using isolated ginsenosides or pure ginsenoside extracts.

It is interesting to note that ginseng will increase serum cortisol levels in nondiabetic individuals but that serum cortisol levels will be reduced in patients with diabetes.[33] Because cortisol, an adrenal hormone, antagonizes insulin, this is presumably a beneficial effect in the diabetic. In addition, the ginseng compound DPG-3-2 exhibits hypoglycemic action or provokes insulin secretion only in diabetic and glucose-loaded normal mice while having no effect on normal mice fed a standard diet.[28] This demonstrates again ginseng's nonspecific balancing effect, baffling to researchers who are accustomed to investigating compounds with consistent pharmacological effects.

Ginseng is indicated as a supportive therapy in the treatment of diabetes, both for its hypoglycemic effect and for its ability to decrease atherosclerosis.

Reproductive effects

Although ginseng is claimed to be a "sexual rejuvenator," human studies supporting this belief are scanty. Ginseng has, however, been shown to promote the growth of the testes and increase sperm formation in rabbits, accelerate the growth of the ovary and enhance ovulation in frogs, stimulate egg-laying in hens, increase gonadal weight in both male and female rats, and increase sexual activity and mating behavior in male rats.[2,34,64] These animal study results seem to support ginseng's use as a fertility and virility aid.

In other experimental animal studies, ginseng has been shown to increase testosterone levels while decreasing prostate weight.[35] This research suggests that ginseng should have favorable effects in the treatment of benign prostatic enlargement; however, no clinical trials have yet been reported.

Ginsenosides have also been shown to exert estrogenlike action on the vaginal epithelium. These results are significant enough to prevent the atrophic vaginal changes associated with postmenopause as well as other menopausal symptoms.[36]

Other therapeutic indications involving the reproductive system (based on historical use and experimental evidence) include decreased sperm counts, testicular atrophy or hypofunction, and other organic causes of male infertility, and ovarian atrophy or hypofunction, absence of menstruation, and other organic causes of female infertility. Note that several reports of breast tenderness have been reported in women taking ginseng.[58,59]

Anticancer properties

Long-term oral administration of ginseng to newborn mice has been shown to reduce the incidence and also inhibit the proliferation of tumors induced by various chemical carcinogens, including DMBA, urethane, and aflatoxin B_1.[37] Ginseng also demonstrates antitumor effects.[28]

Cell proliferating and antiaging effects

Ginseng has a dual effect on cell growth: it stimulates cell division in an adequate nutritional environment, but it acts to inhibit cell growth under adverse conditions.[39] Furthermore, ginseng has yielded impressive results in lengthening the life span of cells in culture.[40]

This enhancement of cellular proliferation and function has been shown on a variety of cell types (epithelial, hepatic, lymphocyte, fibroblast, thymic, neural, etc.) and may be a result of potentiation of nerve growth factor (NGF) by ginsenosides.[3,41] NGF levels typically decline with age. These results indicate a potential use of ginseng in healing virtually all tissue types as well as inhibiting the aging process.

Immunostimulating effects

Ginseng possesses immunostimulating activity, as evidenced by its ability to enhance antibody response, cell-mediated immunity, natural killer cell activity, the production of interferon, and lymphocyte and reticuloendothelial system proliferative and phagocytic functions.[42,43] Ginseng has been shown to prevent viral infections in experimental animals,[44] presumably a result of the combination of these effects.

Perhaps the most important of ginseng's immune-enhancing effects is its ability to enhance the activity of the cells of the reticuloendothelial system. This system is composed of white blood cells known as macrophages, which filter the blood and lymph by engulfing and destroying bacteria, viruses, worn-out red blood cells, and other particulate waste matter. Macrophages are found in highest concentrations in the liver, spleen, and lymph nodes. Ginseng stimulates these cells, increasing host defense capacity immensely.

Note that large dosages of ginseng should not be used during an acute infection because of a possible inhibition of some immune functions at high concentrations.[42,45,46] The chronic ingestion of ginseng by individuals with mild immune deficiency (evidenced by frequent colds) may reduce the risk of viral infection. Use in this manner is consistent with the historical use of ginseng by debilitated individuals.

Cardiovascular effects

Ginseng has paradoxical effects on blood pressure. It appears that at low doses it possesses a hypertensive, or blood pressure increasing, effect, but when administered in larger doses, a hypotensive, or blood pressure lowering, effect is noted.[47] Accordingly, it has been reported useful in the treatment of high blood pressure in humans, but it has also been shown to have blood pressure raising effects as well.[48] This latter effect must be kept in mind when administering ginseng to both normotensive and hypertensive individuals.

Ginseng administered to human subjects with hyperlipidemia (elevated lipids or fats in the blood) has been shown to reduce total serum cholesterol, triglyceride, and fatty acid levels, while raising serum HDL-cholesterol levels (HDL-cholesterol has been shown to actually protect against atherosclerosis). Platelet adhesiveness was also decreased.[49]

These results in humans confirmed earlier studies on rats that were fed high-cholesterol diets.[50,51] The mechanism of action appears to be through accelerated degradation, conversion, and excretion of cholesterol and triglyceride.

From a clinical perspective, it appears that ginseng may offer some protection against atherosclerotic disease, further supporting its use as a general tonic. It also may have a blood pressure regulating effect and reduce excessive blood clot formation.[63]

Liver effects

Obviously, any adaptogenic substance must impact the liver, due to the liver's central role in metabolic and detoxification reactions. Ginseng affects the liver in several ways. As was previously mentioned, ginseng enhances the activity of macrophages. The liver has specialized macrophages known as Kupffer cells.[4,19] Because these cells are responsible for filtering out much of the toxins and debris from the circulation, increasing their activity could have profound effect.

Ginseng has also been shown to increase protein synthesis in the liver.[3,52,53,54] Protein synthesis is often reduced in the elderly, so the significance of the above described effects on enhancement of hepatic protein synthesis would be extremely beneficial. However, these results have yet to be confirmed by clinical studies.

Ginseng has also been shown to reverse diet-induced fatty liver in animals and to possess significant protection to the liver against damage by chemicals.[49,55] The clinical indications of these hepatic actions of ginseng are quite broad and support its general tonic/adaptogen properties.

Radiation protecting effects

Ginseng has been shown to offer some protection against harmful radiation and to hasten recovery from radiation sickness.[56,57] In wake of ever-increasing environmental radiation contamination, ginseng use may be an appropriate preventive measure.

Summary

The therapeutic applications of ginseng are quite broad because of its adaptogenic qualities. Ginseng could be used as a general tonic, especially in debilitated and feeble individuals or whenever fatigue or lack of vigilance is apparent; it can be used to increase mental and physical performance, to prevent the negative effects of stress and enhance the body's response to stress; to offset the negative effects of cortisone, to prevent against atherosclerosis by lowering cholesterol levels, to enhance liver function, and to protect against radiation damage. Ginseng can be used as a supportive therapy in the treatment of diabetes; in conditions involving the reproductive system, including decreased sperm counts, testicular atrophy or hypofunction, and other organic causes of male infertility, and ovarian atrophy or hypofunction, absence of menstruation, and other organic causes of female infertility.

Dosage

The dosage of ginseng is related to the ginsenoside content; i.e., if an extract or ginseng preparation contains high concentrations of ginsenosides (and presumably other active components), a lower dose will suffice.

Currently, there is almost a total lack of quality control in ginseng products marketed in the United States. Independent research and published studies have clearly documented that there is a tremendous variation in the ginsenoside content of commercial preparations.[3,4] In fact, the majority of products on the market contain only trace amounts of ginsenosides, and many formulations contain no ginseng at all. This has led to several problems, ranging from toxicity reactions[60] to lack of medicinal effect. The widespread disregard for quality control in the health food industry has done much to tarnish the reputation of ginseng as well as other important botanicals.

The use of standardized ginseng preparations is recommended to ensure sufficient ginsenoside content, consistent therapeutic results, and reduced risk of toxicity. Products should be standardized by their ginsenoside content. The typical dose (taken one to three times daily) for general tonic effects should contain a saponin content of at least 25 mg of ginsenoside R_{g1} with a ratio R_{g1} to R_{b1} of 2:1. For example, for a high-quality ginseng root powder containing 5% ginsenosides, the dose would be 500 mg; for a standardized *Panax ginseng* extract containing an 18% saponin content calculated as ginsenoside R_{g1}, the standard dose would be 150 mg. The standard dose for high-quality ginseng root is in the range of 4–6 g daily.

Because each individual's response to ginseng is unique, users must take care to observe possible ginseng toxicity. It is best to begin at lower doses and increase gradually. The Russian approach for long-term administration is to use ginseng cyclically for a period of 15–20 days followed by a 2-week interval without any ginseng.

Toxicology

The problem of quality control makes toxicology difficult to address. A 1979 JAMA article titled "Ginseng abuse syndrome" reported a number of side effects, including hypertension, euphoria, nervousness, insomnia, skin eruptions, and morning diarrhea.[60]

Given the extreme variation in quality of ginseng in the American marketplace and the use both of nonofficial parts of the plant and of adulterants, it is not surprising that side effects were noted. None of the commercial preparations used in the trial had been subjected to controlled analysis. Furthermore, the species of ginseng used included *Panax ginseng, P. quinquefolium, Eleutherococcus senticosus,* and *Rumex hymenosepalus* in a variety of different forms, i.e., roots, capsules, tablets, teas, extracts, cigarettes, chewing gum, and candies.

It is virtually impossible to derive any firm conclusions from the data presented in the JAMA article. The author's final words, however, do seem sensible and appropriate: "An important caveat is that these GAS (ginseng abuse syndrome) effects are neither uniformly negative nor uniformly predictable. Nevertheless, long-term ingestion of large amounts of ginseng should be avoided, as even a panacea can cause problems if abused."

Studies performed on standardized extracts of ginseng have demonstrated the absence of side effects as well as the absence of mutagenic or teratogenic effects.[4,12,61,62]

References

1. Leung AY: Encyclopedia of Common Natural Ingredients Used in Food, Drugs and Cosmetics. John Wiley & Sons, New York, NY, 1980. pp186-9
2. Shibata S, Tanaka O, Shoji J, and Saito H: Chemistry and pharmacology of Panax. Economic and Medicinal Plant Research 1:217-84, 1985
3. Liberti LE and Marderosian AD: Evaluation of commercial ginseng products. J Pharm Sci 67:1487-9, 1978
4. Bombardelli E: Ginseng: chemical, pharmacological, and clinical profile. Monograph from Indena S.p.A., Milan, Italy
5. Duke JA: Handbook of Medicinal Herbs. CRC Press, Boca Raton, FL, 1985. pp337-8
6. Brekhman II and Dardymov IV: New substances of plant origin which increase nonspecific resistance. Ann Rev Pharmacol 9:419-30, 1969
7. Brekhman II and Dardymov IV: Pharmacological investigation of glycosides from ginseng and Eleutherococcus. Lloydia 32:46-51, 1969
8. Petkov W: Pharmacological studies of the drug P. ginseng C.A. Meyer. Arzniem Forsch 9:305-11, 1959
9. Petkov W: The mechanism of action of P. ginseng. Arzniem Forsch 11:288-95, 418-22, 1961
10. Petkov W: Effect of ginseng on the brain biogenic monoamines and 3',5'-AMP system. Experiments in rats. Arzniem Forsch 28:388-93, 1978
11. Saito H, Yoshida Y and Takagi K: Effect of Panax ginseng root on exhaustive exercise in mice. Jap J Pharmacol 24:119-27, 1974
12. Kaku T, Miyata T, Uruno T, et al: Chemicopharmacological studies on saponins of Panax ginseng C.A. Meyer. Arzniem Forsch 25:539-47, 1975
13. Avakia EV and Evonuk E: Effects of Panax ginseng extract on tissue glycogen and adrenal cholesterol depletion during prolonged exercise. Planta Medica 36:43-8, 1979
14. Sterner W and Kirchdorfer AM: Comparative work load tests on mice with standardized ginseng extract and a ginseng containing pharmaceutical preparation. Z Gerontol 3:307-12, 1970
15. Hong SA, Park CW, Kim JH, et al: The effects of ginseng saponin on animal behavior. Proceedings of the 1st International Ginseng Symposium, 1975. pp33-44
16. Samira MMH, Attia MA, Allam M and Elwan O: Effect of the standardized ginseng extract G115 on the metabolism and electrical activity of the rabbit's brain. J Int Med Res 13:342-8, 1985
17. Hallstrom C, Fulder S and Carruthers M: Effect of ginseng on the performance of nurses on night duty. Comp Med East & West 6:277-82, 1982
18. D'Angelo L, Grimaldi R, Caravaggi M, et al: A double-blind, placebo controlled clinical study on the effect of a standardized ginseng extract on psychomotor performance in healthy volunteers. J Ethnopharmacol 16:15-22, 1986

19. Bombardelli E, Cirstoni A and Lietti A: The effect of acute and chronic (Panax) ginseng saponins treatment on adrenal function; biochemical and pharmacological. Proceedings 3rd International Ginseng Symposium, 1980, p9-16
20. Fulder SJ: Ginseng and the hypothalamic-pituitary control of stress. Am J Chin Med 9:112-8, 1981
21. Hiai S, Yokoyama H and Oura H: Features of ginseng saponin-induced corticosterone secretion. Endocrinol Japan 26:737-40, 1979
22. Hiai S, Yokoyama H, Oura H, and Kawashima Y: Evaluation of corticosterone secretion-inducing effects of ginsenosides and their prosapogenins and sapogenins. Chem Pharm Bull 31:168-74, 1983
23. Tanizawa H, Numano H, Odani T, et al: Study of the saponin of P. ginseng C.A. Meyer. I. Inhibitory effect on adrenal atrophy, thymus atrophy and the decrease of serum potassium ion concentration induced by cortisone acetate in unilaterally adrenalectomized rats. J Pharm Soc Jap 101:169-73, 1981
24. Hiai S, Yokoyama H, Nagasawa T, and Oura H: Stimulation of the pituitary-adrenocortical axis by saikosaponin of Bupleuri Radix. Chem Pharm Bull 29:495-9, 1981
25. See Chapter 21 Licorice.
26. See Chapter 4 Turmeric
27. Farnsworth NR, Kinghorn AD, Soejarto DD, and Waller DP: Siberian ginseng (Eleutherococcus senticosus): current status as an adaptogen. Economic and Medicinal Plant Research 1:156-215, 1985
28. NG TB and Yeung HW: Hypoglycemic constituents of Panax ginseng. Gen Pharmacol 6:549-552, 1985
29. Waki I, Kyo H, Yasuda M, and Kimura M: effects of a hypoglycemic component of ginseng radix on insulin biosynthesis in normal and diabetic animals. J Pharm Dyn 5:547-54, 1982
30. Konno C, Sugiyama K, Kano M, et al: Isolation and hypoglycaemic activity of panaxans A, B, C, D and E, glycans of Panax ginseng roots. Planta Medica 51:434-6, 1984
31. Kimura M, Waki I, Tanaka O, et al: Pharmacological sequential trials for the fractionation of components with hypoglycemic activity in alloxan diabetic mice from ginseng radix. J Pharm Dyn 4:402-9, 1981
32. Kimura M, Waki I, Tanaka O, et al: Effects of hypoglycemic components in ginseng radix on blood insulin level in alloxan diabetic mice and on insulin release from perfused rat pancreas. J Pharm Dyn 4:410-7, 1981
33. Yamamoto M and Uemura T: Endocrinological and metabolic actions of P. ginseng principles. Proceeding 3rd International Ginseng Symposium, 1980, pp115-9
34. Kim C, Choi H, Kim CC, et al: Influence of ginseng on mating behavior of male rats. Am J Chinese Med 4:163-8, 1976
35. Fahim WS, Harman JM, Clevenger TE, et al: Effect of Panax ginseng on testosterone level and prostate in male rats. Arch Androl 8:261-3, 1982
36. Punnonen R and Lukola A: Oestrogen-like effect of ginseng. Br Med J 281:1110, 1980
37. Yun TK, Yun YS and Han IW: Anticarcinogenic effect of long-term oral administration of newborn mice exposed to various chemical carcinogens. Cancer Detect Prevent 6:515-25, 1983
38. Lee KD and Huemer RP: Antitumoral activity of Panax ginseng extracts. Jap J Pharmacol 21:299-302, 1971
39. Fulder SJ: The growth of cultured human fibroblasts treated with hydrocortisone and extracts of the medicinal plant Panax ginseng. Exp Gerontol 12:125-31, 1977
40. Saito H: Ginsenoside-Rb1 and nerve growth factor (P. ginseng). Proceeding 3rd International Ginseng Symposium, 1981, pp181-5
41. Yamamoto M, Masaka K, Yamada Y, et al: Stimulatory effect of ginsenosides on DNA, protein and lipid synthesis in bone marrow. Arzneim Forsch 28:2238-41, 1978
42. Jie YH, Cammisuli S and Baggiolini M: Immunomodulatory effects of Panax ginseng C.A. Meyer in the mouse. Agents and actions 15:386-91, 1984
43. Gupta S, Agarwal LB, Epstein G, et al: Panax: a new mitogen and interferon producer. Clin Res 28:504A, 1980
44. Singh VK, Agarwal SS and Gupta BM: Immunomodulatory activity of Panax ginseng extract. Planta Medica 51:462-5, 1984
45. Chong SKF, Brown HA, Rimmer E, et al: In vitro effect of Panax ginseng on phytohaemagglutinin-induced lymphocyte transformation. Int Arch Allergy Appl Immun 73:216-20, 1984
46. Yeung HW, Cheung K and Leung KN: Immunopharmacology of Chinese medicine. I. Ginseng induced immunosuppression in virus infected mice. Am J Chin Med 10:44-54, 1982
47. Oh JS, Lim JK, Park CW, and Han MH: The effect of ginseng on experimental hypertension. Korean J Pharmacol 4:27-31, 1968
48. Siegel RK: Ginseng and high blood pressure (letter). JAMA 243:32, 1980
49. Yamamoto M, Uemura T, Nakama S, et al: Serum HDL-cholesterol-increasing and fatty liver-improving action of Panax ginseng in high cholesterol diet-fed rats with clinical effect on hyperlipidemia in man. Am J Chin Med 11:96-101, 1983

50. Yamamoto M and Kumagai: Plasma lipid lowering actions of ginseng saponins and mechanisms of the action. Am J Chin Med 11:84-7, 1983
51. Joo CN: The preventative effect of Korean (P. ginseng) saponins on aortic atheroma formation in prolonged cholesterol-fed rabbits. Proceeding 3rd International Ginseng Symposium, 1980, pp27-36
52. Oura H, Hiai S and Seno H: Synthesis and characterization of nuclear RNA induced by Radix ginseng extract in rat liver. Chem Pharm Bull 19:1598-1605, 1971
53. Oura H, Hiai S, Nabatini S, Nakagawa H, et al: Effect on ginseng on endoplasmic reticulum and ribosome. Planta Medica 28:76-88, 1975
54. Oura H, Nakashima S, Tsukada K, and Ohta Y: Effect of radix ginseng on serum protein synthesis. Chem Pharm Bull 20:980-6, 1972
55. Hikino H, Kiso Y, Sanada S, and Shoji J: Antihepatotoxic actions of ginsenosides from Panax ginseng roots. Planta Medica 52:62-4, 1985
56. Ben-Hur E and Fulder S: Effect of P. ginseng saponins and Eleutherococcus S. on survival of cultured mammalian cells after ionizing radiation. Am J Chin Med 9:48-56, 1981
57. Yonezawa M: Restoration of radiation injury by intraperitoneal injection of ginseng extract in mice. J Radiation Res 17:111-3, 1976
58. Palmer BV, Montgomery ACV and Monteiro JCMP: Ginseng and mastalgia (letter). Br Med J i:1284, 1978
59. Koriech OM: Ginseng and mastalgia (letter). Br Med J i:1556, 1978
60. Siegel RK: Ginseng abuse syndrome. JAMA 241:1614-5, 1979
61. Hess FG, Parent RA, Cox GE, et al: Effects of subchronic feeding of ginsenoside extract G115 in beagle dogs. Food Chem Toxicol 21:95-7, 1983
62. Hess FG, Parent RA, Cox GE, et al: Reproduction study in rats of ginseng extract G115. Food Chem Toxicol 20:189, 1982
63. Matsuda H, Namba K, Fukuda S, et al: Pharmacological study on Panax ginseng C.A. Meyer III Effects of red ginseng on experimental disseminated intravascular coagulation. (2). Effects of ginsenosides on blood coagulative and fibrinolytic systems. Chem Pharm Bull 34:1153-7, 1986
64. Yamamoto M, Kumagai A and Yamamura Y: Stimulatory effect of P. ginseng principles on DNA and protein synthesis in rat testes. Arzneim Forsch 27:1404-5, 1977
65. Minmo Y, Ota N, Sakao S, and Shimomura S: Determination of germanium in medicinal plants by atomic absorption spectrometry with electrothermal atomization. Chem Pharm Bull 28:2687-91, 1980

6

Siberian ginseng
(ELEUTHEROCOCCUS SENTICOSUS)

Key uses of Siberian ginseng:

- Stress and fatigue
- Atherosclerosis
- Performance enhancement
- Impaired kidney function

General description

Eleutherococcus senticosus, or Siberian ginseng, is a shrub, usually 1.5–2.6 m high, with erect, spiny shoots and light gray or brownish bark and a trunk 4–6 cm in diameter. The leaves are long-petioled in a compound palmate configuration. The leaflets (five) are elliptic and finely serrated at the margins on both sides and have scattered, minute spinules along the veins.[1,2]

Siberian ginseng grows abundantly in parts of the Soviet Far East, Korea, China, and Japan, north of latitude 38. Its distribution is actually much greater than that of *Panax ginseng*.[1]

The root is the most widely used medicinal part. The highest concentration of biologically active substances in the root occur in the fall, just before defoliation. The leaves are also used medicinally. The highest concentration of biologically active substances in the leaves occur in July, just before flowering.

Chemical composition

The initial chemical report on Siberian ginseng, also known as eleuthero, was published in 1965 by members of the Institute of Biologically Active Substances, in Vladivostok, U.S.S.R.[1] Seven compounds, termed eleutherosides A–G, were isolated from a physiologically active fraction of the methanol extract of eleuthero. The total eleutheroside content of the root is in the range of 0.6–0.9%; eleutheroside content in the stems is in the range of 0.6–1.5%. Thin-layer chromatographic analysis has shown that the ginsenoside characteristics of *Panax* sp. (American, Chinese, Korean, Japanese ginsengs) are not present in the roots of *E. senticosus*.

History and folk use

The ginseng plants—i.e., members of the family Araliaceae, including *E. senticosus*—are among the most honored and ancient of all medicinal herbs. Their use in Chinese herbal medicine dates back more than 4,000 years.[1-3] Confusion has arisen at times over the lack of specificity in ancient documents in regard to exactly what member of the ginseng family was being referred to. However, the value of eleuthero as a medicinal agent was certainly known to the Chinese, as evidenced by the following Chinese ode to wujia (*E. senticosus*):

ODE TO WUJIA
by Ye Zhishen (Qing Dynasty)
From earth and heavens the quintessence originates,
Five folioles clustering your leaves,
And pretty little thorns wrapped whole your shoots;
Oh what a jackal's gaunt leg looks much alike.
How wonderful is Winzhang-grass, the Eleuthero-ginseng
Dispensing in liquor for drinking,
And decocting with burnet for daily using;
It will keep your virgin face younger
And prolong your life for ever and ever;
Even if a cartload of gold and jewels,
That can not estimate your price of nature.[3]

In summary, the Chinese believe that the regular use of eleuthero will increase longevity, improve general health, improve the appetite, and restore memory.

Despite a long history of use by Chinese herbalists (references date back to 2000 B.C.), the Russians have a separate history of eleuthero and even go so far as to say, "Eleutherococcus was not known in Oriental folk medicine."[1] The Russian history of eleuthero begins in 1855 when a pair of Russian scientists, C. I. Maximovich and L. I. Shrenk, traveled from St. Petersburg (now Leningrad) to the Ussuri region of Russia on the Amur river. It was in this area that Maximovich observed a vast thicket of unusual plants with leaves resembling those of the horse chestnut and with young shoots resembling those of ginseng. Unable to identify the plant, the two scientists returned to St. Petersburg with the plant for classification. The plant was given the genus name of *Eleuthero* or "free-berried shrub" and the species name of *senticosus*, which means "thorny" in Latin.

Eleuthero remained largely unknown to Russians for roughly 100 years after Maximovich's discovery. It wasn't until the middle of the 20th century that eleuthero was "discovered" when Russian scientists began investigating substances that produce a "state of nonspecific resistance" on the body. Substances having this effect were termed adaptogens. As defined by Brekhman in 1958, an adaptogen is a substance that: (1) must be innocuous and cause minimal disorders in the physiological functions of an organism; (2) must have a nonspecific action (i.e., it should increase the resistance to adverse influences by a wide range of physical, chemical, and biochemical factors); and (3) usually has a normalizing action irrespective of the direction of the pathologic state (alterative action).[1,4]

Brekhman's research with adaptogens began with *Panax ginseng* since this was the best known natural adaptogen. After confirming this adaptogenic action of ginseng in human studies, Brekhman began searching for an alternative to this plant because of the difficulty in obtaining ginseng and its expense. Initially, all six species of Araliaceae native to Russia were investigated, but eleuthero appeared to be the most promising. Numerous studies have been done on eleuthero since the late 1950s, with the overwhelming majority being conducted in the Soviet Union.[1-8]

Pharmacology

As mentioned, a number of experimental and clinical studies have demonstrated that eleuthero does possess adaptogenic properties; i.e., the ability to increase nonspecific body resistance to stress, fatigue, and disease. Further experimental and clinical research supports additional therapeutic applications of *Eleutherococcus senticosus*.

Adaptogenic activity

An important characteristic of an adaptogen is its ability to "normalize" irrespective of the direction of pathology. *E. senticosus* has been shown in experimental models to do just this.[1-7] Similar results have been obtained with *P. ginseng*.

Another important action of adaptogens is to inhibit the alarm phase (fight or flight response) of the stress reaction. Eleuthero has shown similar action to *P. ginseng* in the experiments designed to demonstrate an antialarm action. Specifically, eleuthero has been shown to increase the swimming time of rats, reduce activation of the adrenal cortex in response to stress (alarm phase reaction), and prevent stress-induced damage to the thymus gland and lymphatic system.[1-7]

In addition to its confirmed adaptogenic activity, eleuthero has also demonstrated a protective and medicinal action in animals exposed to both single and prolonged X-ray radiation. In one study, both *E. senticosus* and *P. ginseng* doubled the life span of rats exposed to prolonged radiation (total doses of 1,620–7,000 rad). When eleuthero was combined with antibiotics, the life span of irradiated rats (exposed for 60 days with a total dose of 3,000 rad) increased threefold.[8]

These results suggest that eleuthero may be of benefit in protecting against harmful radiation and as an aid in radiation therapy in cancer patients. The latter suggestion is further supported by studies of eleuthero that have demonstrated an inhibition of cancer.[1,4]

It is evident from the discussion of eleuthero's adaptogenic activities that eleuthero shares many features with *P. ginseng*. In addition to the adaptogenic activities discussed, eleuthero, like panax, has been shown to increase resistance to infection in animals, reduce cholesterol biosynthesis in the liver, increase reproductive capacity and sperm counts in bulls, possess significant antioxidant activity, and stimulate protein synthesis and cellular repair enzymes.[1]

Eleuthero as an adaptogen in
normal and stressed individuals

Farnsworth and colleagues have reviewed data on an *E. senticosus* root extract (33% ethanol) administered to more than 2,100 healthy human subjects in clinical trials for the purpose of evaluating the adaptogenic effects of eleuthero.[1] These studies indicated that eleuthero: (1) increased the ability of humans to withstand many adverse physical conditions (i.e., heat, noise, motion, workload increase, exercise, and decompression), (2) increased mental alertness and work output, and (3) improved the quality of work under stressful conditions and athletic performance.

The studies were composed of both male and female subjects ranging from 19 to 72 years old. Doses of the 33% ethanol (fluid) extract of *E. senticosus* roots ranged from 2.0–16.0 ml, one to three times a day, for periods of up to 60 consecutive days. In multiple dosing regimens, there is usually a 2- to 3-week interval between courses.

Eleuthero as an adaptogen in disease processes

Farnsworth et al. have also reviewed data on an *E. senticosus* root extract (33% ethanol) administered to more than 2,200 human subjects in clinical trials for the purpose of evaluating the adaptogenic effects of eleuthero in disease states.[1] A variety of illnesses were included in these studies, including angina, hypertension, hypotension, acute pyleonephritis, various types of neuroses, acute craniocerebral trauma, rheumatic heart disease, chronic bronchitis, and cancer.

Eleuthero appears to be effective in atherosclerotic conditions, as evidenced by its ability to lower elevated serum cholesterol, reduce blood pressure, and eliminate angina symptoms in human subjects. Its action on blood pressure is truly adaptogenic because eleuthero has also been shown to increase blood pressure in subjects who have low blood pressure.[1]

Its affect in regulating blood pressure may indicate improved kidney function. Patients with acute kidney infection who were given eleuthero extract demonstrated improved kidney function.[1]

Eleuthero appears to have some action on the brain as well. It was shown to be effective in the treatment of a variety of psychological disturbances. Consistently, eleuthero has demonstrated an ability to increase the sense of well-being regardless of the psychological complaint (insomnia, hypochondriasis, various neuroses, etc.). A possible explanation of this effect is improved balance between the various biogenic amines (serotonin, dopamine, norepinephrine, epinephrine, etc.) that act as transmitters in the nervous system. Eleuthero extract administered to rats has been shown to increase biogenic amine content in the brain, adrenals, and urine.[1]

There is insufficient data to fully evaluate eleuthero's action on other disease states at this time. However, it must be kept in mind that an adaptogen must be nonspecific in its action and possess a normalizing action irrespective of the direction of the changes from physiological norms.

Summary

E. senticosus, or Siberian ginseng, possesses significant adaptogenic action. Currently, its use can be recommended as a general tonic and in some clinical situations (angina, hypertension, hypotension, kidney infection, various types of psychological complaints, rheumatic heart disease, chronic bronchitis, and cancer). It must be pointed out, however, that clinical applications of Siberian ginseng may be much greater due to its nonspecific mechanisms of action.

Dosage

The standard dosage of the 33% ethanol extract (fluid extract) of *E. senticosus* roots used in the majority of studies ranged from 2.0–4.0 ml (up to 16.0 ml), one to three times a day, for periods of up to 60 consecutive days. In multiple dosing regimens, there is usually a 2- to 3-week interval between courses.[1,4] Dosages three times a day are as follows:

- Dried root—2–4 g
- Tincture (1:5)—10–20 ml (2½–5 tsp)
- Fluid extract (1:1)—2.0–4.0 ml (½–1 tsp)
- Solid (dry, powdered) extract (20:1, containing greater than 1% eleutheroside E)—100–200 mg

Toxicology

Toxicity studies in animals have demonstrated that eleuthero extracts are virtually nontoxic. The LD_{50} of the 33% ethanol extract of eleuthero is 14.5 ml/kg in mice and greater than 20.0 ml/kg in rats. No long-term toxicity was observed in rats administered the 33% ethanol extract of eleuthero at a daily dose of 5.0 ml/kg.[1]

In human studies, it was demonstrated that Eleuthero extracts (33% ethanol) are extremely well tolerated and side effects are extremely infrequent. However, side effects are often reported at higher dosages (4.5–6.0 ml three times a day). Side effects include insomnia, irritability, melancholy, and anxiety. In individuals with rheumatic heart disease, pericardial pain, headaches, palpitations, and elevations in blood pressure have been reported.[1]

References

1. Farnsworth NR, Kinghorn AD, Soejarto D and Waller DP: Siberian ginseng (Eleutherococcus senticosus): Current status as an adaptogen. Economic Medicinal Plant Research 1:156-215, 1985
2. Leung AY: Encyclopedia of Common Natural Ingredients Used in Food, Drugs and Cosmetics. John Wiley & Sons, New York, NY 1980 pp186-9
3. Duke JA: Handbook of Medicinal Herbs. CRC Press, Boca Raton, FL 1985 pp337-8
4. Baranov AI: Medicinal uses of ginseng and related plants in the Soviet Union: Recent trends in the Soviet literature. J Ethnopharmacol 6:339-53, 1982
5. Brekhman II and Dardymov IV: New substances of plant origin which increase nonspecific resistance. Annual Rev Pharmacol 9:419-30, 1969
6. Brekhman II and Dardymov IV: Pharmacological investigation of glycosides from ginseng and Eleutherococcus. Lloydia 32:46-51, 1969
7. Brekhman II and Kirillov OI: Effect of Eleutherococcus on alarm-phase of stress. 8:113-121, 1969
8. Ben-Hur E and Fulder S: Effect of P. ginseng saponins and Eleutherococcus S. on survival of cultured mammalian cells after ionizing radiation. Am J Chinese Med 9:48-56, 1981

7

Angelica *species*

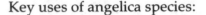

Key uses of angelica species:

- Menopausal symptoms
- Premenstrual syndrome
- Allergies
- Smooth muscle spasm

Angelica sinensis or *polymorpha* (family Umbelliferae or Apiaceae)
  Common names: Chinese angelica, dong quai
Angelica acutiloba (family Umbelliferae or Apiaceae)
  Common name: Japanese angelica
Angelica archangelica (family Umbelliferae or Apiaceae)
  Common name: European angelica
Angelica atropurpurea (family Umbelliferae or Apiaceae)
  Common name: American angelica
Angelica sylvestris (family Umbelliferae or Apiaceae)
  Common name: Wild angelica

General description

Angelica species are biennial or perennial plants with hollow, fluted stems
that rise to a height of 3–7 feet. Greenish-white flowers bloom from May to
August. The plants are found in damp mountain ravines and meadows, on
river banks, and in coastal areas; angelica is also a widely cultivated species.
In Asia, it is grown primarily for its medicinal action. In the United States and
Europe, angelica is cultivated for use as a flavoring agent in most major
categories of food products, including nonalcoholic and alcoholic beverages
(e.g., bitters, liqueurs, and vermouths), ice cream, candy, gelatin, and pud-
dings. With all species, the roots and rhizomes are the most extensively used
portions of the plant.

Angelica sinensis and A. acutiloba

In Asia, the authentic and original medicinal angelica is *Angelica sinensis* (dong quai), native to China. Although at least nine other angelica species are used in China, dong quai is by far the most highly regarded. For several thousand years, dong quai has been cultivated for medicinal use in the treatment of a wide variety of disorders—in particular, "female" disorders. It is often referred to as the "female ginseng."

Several hundred years ago, when the supply of Chinese angelica was scarce, the Japanese began to cultivate *A. acutiloba*, an angelica species indigenous to Japan, as a substitute.[1] The two species appear to have very similar therapeutic effects, although it is interesting to note that in China, the Japanese angelica is thought to have no therapeutic value; in Japan, Chinese angelica is thought to have no effect. Experimentally, both species exhibit very similar therapeutic effects, and each country's claim to produce a superior dong quai is based more on emotion than scientific investigation.

Angelica archangelica and A. atropurpurea

Historical usage suggests that European angelica (*A. archangelica*) and American angelica (*A. atropurpurea*) have properties different from the Asian species. This difference has not, however, been evaluated by chemical analysis.

Chemical composition

Angelica sinensis and A. acutiloba

No comprehensive data could be found listing the concentration of the chemical constituents. It is assumed that Chinese and Japanese angelica are similarly composed of various coumarins and flavonoids responsible for their medicinal actions. The essential oil of Oriental angelica contains *n*-butylphthalide, cadinene, carvacrol, *n*-dodecanal, isosafrole, linoleic acid, palmitic acid, safrole, sequiterpene, and *n*-tetradecanol.[2]

Angelica archangelica

Also very rich in coumarins, this species of angelica is particularly phototoxic. Coumarins, including osthole, angelicin, osthenol, umbelliferone, archangelicine, bergapten, and ostruthol, are found in significant concentrations, with osthole composing nearly 0.2% of the root. The root is also a good source of flavonoids, including archangelenone and caffeic acids. The root contains 0.3–1.0% volatile oil that is composed mainly of beta-phyllamdrene, alpha-pinene, borneol, limonene, and four macrocylic lactones.[2,3]

History and folk use

Angelica sinensis and A. acutiloba

In Asia, angelica's reputation is perhaps second only to ginseng. Predominantly regarded as a "female" remedy, angelica has been used in such conditions as dysmenorrhea (painful menstruation), amenorrhea (absence of menstruation), metrorrhagia (abnormal menstruation), and menopausal symptoms (especially hot flashes). It also has been used to assure a healthy pregnancy and easy delivery. Angelica is also used in the treatment of abdominal pain, anemia, injuries, arthritis, migraine headache, and many other conditions.[2,4]

Angelica archangelica

One of the most highly praised herbs in old herbal texts, archangelica was used by all North European countries as:

> a protection against contagion, for purifying the blood, and for curing every conceivable malady: it was held a sovereign remedy for poisons, agues and all infectious maladies.

According to one legend, archangelica was revealed in a dream as a cure for the plague. One explanation for the name is related to its blooming near May 8, the feast day of Michael the Archangel. It was therefore seen as a "protector against evil spirits and witchcraft."[6]

Archangelica has been used for a wide variety of conditions, including flatulent dyspepsia, pleurisy, respiratory catarrh, and bronchitis. The plant was believed to possess carminative, spasmolytic, diaphoretic, expectorant, and diuretic activity.[6]

Angelica atropurpurea

American angelica's therapeutic use mirrors that of European angelica. Its most common use is for heartburn and flatulent colic.[7]

Pharmacology

The pharmacology of *Angelica* sp. relates to their high coumarin content. However, unlike other scientific investigations of botanical medicines, much of the research done on *Angelica* sp. has been done on plant extracts, rather than with isolated constituents. The overwhelming majority of the studies has been done on the Asian species. Some of the pharmacological activities demonstrated include phytoestrogen activity, analgesic activity, cardiovascular effects, smooth muscle relaxing effects, antiallergy and immunomodulating activity, and antibacterial activity.

Phytoestrogen effects

Plant estrogenic substances or phytoestrogens are components of many medicinal herbs with an historic use in conditions that are now treated by synthetic estrogens. Chinese and Japanese angelica contain highly active phytoestrogens, although these compounds are much lower in activity than animal estrogens (1:400 as active), which helps explain why angelica was used in both conditions of high and low estrogens. Phytoestrogens demonstrate an alterative effect by competing with estrogen for binding sites. When estrogen levels are low, they are able to exert some estrogenic activity; when the estrogen levels are high, they reduce overall estrogenic activity by occupying estrogen receptor sites. This alterative action of angelica's phytoestrogens is most likely the basis of much of the plant's use in amenorrhea and menopause.

Japanese angelica has demonstrated uterine tonic activity, causing an initial increase in uterine contraction followed by relaxation.[8,9] Administering Japanese angelica to mice resulted in an increase of uterine weight, an increase of the DNA content of the uterus and liver, and an increase of glucose utilization by the liver and uterus.[1,8] Because of these and other effects, angelica has been referred to as a uterine tonic.

Cardiovascular effects

Although angelica has not been used historically for cardiovascular purposes, it does possess significant hypotensive action,[1,8] largely due to its ability to dilate blood vessels. Dihydropyranocoumarins and dihydrofuranocoumarins from Umbelliferous plants like angelica have been shown to possess significant ability to dilate coronary vessels and relieve vasospasmsasodilatory.[10] The mechanism of action appears to be largely a result of calcium-channel antagonism. Agents that interact with calcium channels (calcium-channel blockers) are quickly coming into prominence in the treatment of a wide variety of conditions, including hypertension and angina. Angelica and other Umbelliferous plants may offer similar effects. Other cardiovascular effects noted for angelica include antiarrhythmic actions.[1]

Smooth muscle relaxing activity

Calcium-channel blocking compounds are also capable of relaxing the smooth muscles of visceral organs. Angelica (essential oil) has demonstrated relaxing action on the smooth muscles of the intestines and uterus, and the water extract produces an initial contraction and then prolonged relaxation.[1,8,9] This confirms angelica's historical use in the treatment of intestinal spasm and uterine cramps. Its action on other smooth muscles could explain its hypotensive action (vascular smooth muscle) and historical use in treating asthma (bronchial smooth muscle).

Analgesic activity

Both Chinese and Japanese angelica have demonstrated pain-relieving and mild tranquilizing effects in experimental studies with animals.[1,8,11,12] Angelica's pain-relieving action was 1.7 times that of aspirin in one study.[12] Its analgesic activity, combined with its smooth muscle relaxing activity, supports its historical use in such conditions as uterine cramps, trauma, headaches, and arthritis.

Antiallergy and immunomodulating activity

Angelica has long been used by Chinese and Japanese herbalists to prevent and treat allergic symptoms in individuals who are sensitive to a variety of substances (pollen, dust, animal dander, food, etc.).[1,13] Its action is related to its ability to inhibit the production of allergic antibodies (IgE) in a selective manner. Since IgE levels in patients with allergic conditions are typically 3 to 10 times greater than the upper limit of normal, angelica may offer some benefit by reducing these elevated antibodies.

Coumarin compounds have demonstrated immune-enhancing activity in both healthy individuals and cancer patients.[14,15] Coumarins have been shown to stimulate white blood cells and increase their ability to destroy foreign particles and cancer cells.[14] Such activity is thought to offer significant protection against the growth and spread of tumor cells. It is said that upon administering coumarin, specific white blood cells known as macrophages are activated and thus are capable of entering the tumor, where they can destroy tumor cells.[14,15]

Coumarin compounds of angelica and the polysaccharides of the water extract of Japanese angelica have immune-modulating activity. They have been shown to increase the activity of white blood cells, increase interferon production, increase antitumor activity, and increase nonspecific host defense mechanisms.[16-19] These effects on the immune system by coumarins, polysaccharides, and extracts of *Angelica* sp. would seem to sustain their historical anticancer effects and their use as support agents to current cancer therapy.

Antibacterial activity

Extracts of Chinese angelica have exhibited antibacterial activity against both gram-negative and gram-positive bacteria, but extracts of Japanese angelica have exhibited no antibacterial action.[8] The inconsistency could be due to different essential oil concentrations of the extracts used in the studies. The oil of *A. archangelica* has exhibited significant antifungal properties but virtually no antibacterial activity.[3,5] Because other herbs have much greater antimicrobial activity, *Angelica* sp. would be considered a less than optimum agent if this effect is desired.

Summary

Angelica sp. have been used throughout the world in the treatment of a wide variety of conditions. At this time it appears that *A. archangelica* and *A. atropurpurea* are most indicated as expectorants, antispasmodics, and carminatives in the treatment of such conditions as respiratory ailments, gas, and abdominal spasm. Chinese angelica (*A. sinensis* or *A. polymorpha*) and Japanese angelica (*A. acutiloba*) appear most useful in the treatment of disorders of menstruation, menopause (especially hot flashes), atopic conditions, smooth muscle spasm (e.g., uterine cramps, migraines, and abdominal spasm), and possibly as an immunostimulatory adjunct in cancer therapy. Further research with human subjects is needed to document the degree of clinical efficacy of *Angelica* sp.

Dosage

The standard dose for the dried root or rhizome of *Angelica* sp. is 1–2 g orally or by infusion three times a day. The dose for the tincture (1:5) is 3–5 ml three times a day, and the fluid extract (1:1) dosage is 0.5–2 ml. For general tonic effects, use doses three times a day.

Toxicology

Angelica is generally considered to be of extremely low toxicity. However, it does contain many photoreactive substances that may induce photosensitivity (reaction to the sun, which usually produces a rash). This warning should be kept in mind when using any Umbelliferous plant. However, the photoreactive substances may actually be therapeutic in the treatment of vitiligo and psoriasis.

References

1. Hikino H: Recent research on Oriental medicinal plants. Economic Medical Plant Research 1:53-85, 1985
2. Duke JA: Handbook of Medicinal Herbs. CRC Press, Boca Raton, FL, 1985. p43-4
3. Leung AY: Encyclopedia of Common Natural Ingredients Used in Food, Drugs, and Cosmetics. John Wiley & Sons. New York, NY, 1980. pp28-9
4. Duke JA and Ayensu ES: Medicinal Plants of China. Reference Publications, Algonac, MI, 1985, pp74-7
5. Opdyke DLJ: Angelica root oil. Food Cosmet Toxicol 13(suppl): 713-4, 1975
6. Grieve M: A Modern Herbal. Dover Publications, New York, NY, 1971. pp35-40
7. Lust J: The Herb Book. Bantam Books, New York, NY, 1974. pp97-99
8. Yoshiro K: The physiological actions of tang-kuei and cnidium. Bull Oriental Healing Arts Inst USA 10:269-78, 1985
9. Harada M, Suzuki M and Ozaki Y: Effect of Japanese angelica root and peony root on uterine contraction in the rabbit in situ. J Pharm Dyn 7:304-11, 1984
10. Thastrup O, Fjalland B and Lemmich J: Coronary vasodilatory, spasmolytic and cAMP-phosphodiesterase inhibitory properties of dihydropyranocoumarins and dihydrofuranocoumarins. Acta Pharmacol et Toxicol 52:246-53, 1983
11. Tanaka S, Ikeshiro Y, Tabata M, and Konoshima M: Anti-nociceptive substances from the roots of Angelica acutiloba. Arzneim Forsch 27:2039-45, 1977
12. Tanaka S, Kano Y, Tabata M and Konoshima M: Effects of "Toki" (Angelica acutiloba Kitawaga) extracts on writhing and capillary permeability in mice (analgesic and anti-inflammatory effects). Yakugaku Zassh 91:1098-1104, 1071
13. Sung CP, Baker AP, Holden DA, et al: Effects of Angelica polymorpha on reaginic antibody production. J Natural Products 45:398-406, 1982
14. Casley-Smith JR: The actions of benzopyrenes on the blood-tissue-lymph system. Folia angiol 24:7-22, 1976
15. Berkarda B, Bouffard-Eyuboglu H and Derman U: The effect of coumarin derivatives on the immunological system of man. Agents Actions 13:50-2, 1983
16. Ohno N, Matsumoto SI, Suzuki I, et al: Biochemical characterization of a mitogen obtained from an oriental crude drug, tohki (Angelica acutiloba Kitawaga). J Pharm Dyn 6:903-12, 1983
17. Yamada H, Kiyohara H, Cyong JC, et al: Studies on polysaccharides from Angelica acutiloba. Planta Medica 48:163-7, 1984
18. Yamada H, Kiyohara H, Cyong JC, et al: Studies on polysaccharides from Angelica acutiloba - IV. Characterization of an anti-complementary arabinogalactan from the roots of Angelica acutiloba Kitagawa. Molecular Immunology 22:295-304, 1985
19. Kumazawa Y, Mizunoe K and Otsuka Y: Immunostimulating polysaccharide separated from hot water extract of Angelica acutiloba Kitagawa (Yamato Tohki). Immunology 47:75-83, 1982

SECTION III

Herbs for liver disorders

The liver is truly an intricate, complex, and remarkable organ. It is, without question, the most important organ of metabolism. To a very large extent, the health and vitality of an individual are determined by the health and vitality of the liver.

It is amazing how well the liver survives the constant onslaught of toxic chemicals it is responsible for detoxifying. Some of the toxic chemicals known to pass through the liver include the polycyclic hydrocarbons that are components of various herbicides and pesticides, including DDT; dioxin; 2,4,5-T; 2,4-D; and the halogenated compounds PCB and PCP. Although the exact degree of exposure of Americans to these compounds is not known, it is probably quite high because yearly production of synthetic organic pesticides alone exceeds 1.4 billion pounds.

The health effects of chronic exposure to these compounds, as well as many others, has not been fully determined (other than the known association with various cancers). Because the liver is responsible for detoxifying these chemicals and many others, every effort should be made to promote optimal liver function.

When the liver is "sluggish" (a condition called cholestasis), individuals may complain of fatigue, general malaise, digestive disturbances, allergies and chemical sensitivities, premenstrual syndrome, and constipation. Presently it appears that clinical judgment based on medical history remains the major diagnostic tool for the sluggish liver. Exposure to toxic chemicals, drugs, alcohol, or hepatitis is usually apparent in the individual with a sluggish liver.

The herbs discussed in this section, milk thistle and dandelion, have remarkable ability to improve and restore liver function. Although there are many herbs that improve liver function, these two herbs stand out.

8

Milk thistle

(SILYBUM MARIANUM)

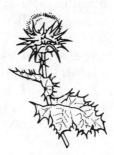

Key uses of milk thistle:

- Liver disorders
- Hepatitis
- Cirrhosis of the liver
- Psoriasis

General description

Silybum marianum, or milk thistle, is a stout, annual or biennial plant found in dry rocky soils in southern and western Europe and some parts of the United States. The branched stem grows 1–3 ft high and bears dark green, shiny leaves with spiny, scalloped edges that are markedly streaked with white along the veins. The solitary flower heads are reddish-purple with bracts ending in sharp spines. Flowering season is from June to August. The seeds, fruit, and leaves are used for medicinal purposes.

Chemical composition

S. marianum contains silymarin, a mixture of flavanolignans, consisting chiefly of silybin, silydianin, and silychristine.[1-3] The concentration of silymarin is highest in the fruit, but it is also found in the seeds and leaves. Silibin is the silymarin component that yields the greatest degree of biological activity.

History and folk use

Perhaps the most widespread folk use of this plant has been in assisting the nursing mother in the production of milk.[10] It was also used in Germany for curing jaundice and biliary derangements.[10] It is interesting to note that the discovery of the liver-protecting compound silymarin in milk thistle was not the result of extensive pharmacological screening but of investigation of silybum's empirical effects in liver disorders.[1]

Pharmacology

S. marianum extracts (usually standardized to contain 70–80% silymarin) are currently widely used in European pharmaceutical preparations for hepatic disorders. Silymarin is one of the most potent liver-protecting substances known.[1-9]

Actions relating to the liver

Milk thistle's ability to prevent liver destruction and enhance liver function is largely a result of silymarin's inhibition of the factors that are responsible for liver damage, coupled with its ability to stimulate the growth of new liver cells to replace old damaged cells. The liver can be damaged as a result of some toxins producing or acting as free radicals. Free radicals are highly reactive molecules that can damage other molecules, including those in cells. Silymarin prevent free radical damage by acting as an antioxidant.[1-4] Silymarin is many times more potent in antioxidant activity than vitamin E. Silymarin has also been shown to increase the glutathione content of the liver by over 35% in healthy subjects. Glutathione is responsible for detoxifying a wide range of hormones, drugs, and chemicals. Increasing the glutathione content of the liver means that the liver has an increased capacity for detoxification reactions.

Another way the liver can be damaged is by the action of leukotrienes. These compounds are produced by the transfer of an oxygen molecule to polyunsaturated fatty acids, a reaction catalyzed by the enzyme lipoxygenase. Silymarin has been shown to be a potent inhibitor of this enzyme, thereby inhibiting the formation of damaging leukotrienes.[12]

Free radical damage to membrane structures from organic disease or intoxication results in increased release of fatty acids. This condition leads to increased leukotriene synthesis and inflammation, among other things. Silymarin counteracts this deleterious process by suppressing the pathological decomposition of membrane lipids and inhibiting leukotriene formation and inflammation.[13]

The protective effect of silymarin against liver damage has been demonstrated in a number of experimental and clinical studies.[1-27] Experimental liver damage in animals can be produced by such diverse toxic chemicals as carbon tetrachloride, galactosamine, ethanol, and praseodymium nitrate. Silymarin has been shown to protect the liver from all these toxins.[1-4,7,34]

Perhaps the most impressive of silymarin's protective effects is against the severe poisoning of *Amanita phalloides* (the deathcap or toadstool mushroom), an effect that has long been recognized in folk medicine.[5-7] Ingestion of *A. phalloides* or its toxins causes severe poisoning and, in approximately 30% of victims, death.

Among the experimental models for measuring protection against liver damage, those based on amanitin or phalloidin toxicity are the most important because these two peptides from *A. phalloides* are the most powerful liver-damaging substances known. Silymarin has demonstrated impressive results in these experimental models. When silymarin was administered before amanita toxin poisoning, it was 100% effective in preventing toxicity.[5,7] Even if given 10 min after the amanita toxin, it completely counteracted the toxic effects. If given within 24 hr, silymarin would still prevent death and greatly reduce the amount of liver damage.[6]

Perhaps the most interesting effect of milk thistle's components on the liver is their ability to stimulate protein synthesis.[4,11,14] This action results in an increase in the production of new liver cells to replace the damaged old ones. Interestingly, silymarin does not have a stimulatory effect on malignant liver tissue.[11] From the hepatic actions described, it is apparent that *S. marianum* and, more specifically, silymarin exerts both a protective and restorative role.

Silymarin in liver disorders

In human studies, silymarin has been shown to have positive effects in treating several types of liver disease, including cirrhosis, chronic hepatitis, fatty infiltration of the liver (chemical- and alcohol-induced fatty liver), subclinical cholestasis of pregnancy, and cholangitis and pericholangitis.[15-27] The therapeutic effect of silymarin in these disorders has been confirmed by histological, clinical, and laboratory data.[15-27]

As mentioned, *S. marianum* and, more specifically, silymarin significantly protects against liver damage by preventing free radical damage and the formation of damaging leukotrienes and by stimulating the production of new liver cells.

In one of the first extensive double-blind clinical trials investigating silymarin's therapeutic effect in liver disorders, silymarin demonstrated impressive results on 129 patients with toxic metabolic liver damage, fatty degeneration of the liver of various origin, or chronic hepatitis, as compared with a control group made up of 56 patients.[15] The results might have been even more impressive if the study had lasted longer than 35 days.

A follow-up study of patients with liver damage due to alcohol, diabetes, viruses, or toxic exposure demonstrated even more striking results. Patients were followed for a long period of time (e.g., 7 weeks). Not only were clinical findings markedly improved in the silymarin-treated groups, but laboratory and liver biopsy data improved as well.[16] Highly significant results were obtained in bromsulphalein retention, SGPT, iron, and cholesterol levels. There were remarkable tissue restorative effects, as biopsies showed. Upon completion of silymarin therapy, the liver showed restitution of normal cell structure in even severely damaged livers. These effects on the tissue level correlated well with improvements in blood chemistry.

The therapeutic effects of silymarin in liver disorders have been duplicated in other double-blind clinical studies.[17-27] Silymarin is particularly effective in protecting against alcohol- and chemical-induced liver damage, and some evidence suggests that it is also of value in viral hepatitis.

Silymarin in psoriasis

Correction of abnormal liver function is indicated in the treatment of psoriasis. Silymarin has been reported to be of value in the treatment of psoriasis, perhaps due to its ability to inhibit the synthesis of leukotrienes and improve liver function.[28,32]

The connection between the liver and psoriasis relates to one of the liver's basic tasks: filtering the blood. Psoriasis has been shown to be linked to high levels of circulating endotoxins, such as those found in the cell walls of gut bacteria. If the liver is overwhelmed by an increased number of endotoxins or chemical toxins, or if the liver's functional ability to filter and detoxify is decreased, the psoriasis gets much worse.

Another factor in psoriasis is excessive production of leukotrienes. Silymarin has been shown to reduce leukotriene formation by inhibiting lipoxygenase.[28] Therefore, silymarin would inhibit one of the causes of the excessive cellular replication.

Silymarin has other effects that would be of value to patients with psoriasis. Most of these effects involve correcting the abnormal cAMP to cGMP ratio observed in the skin of patients with psoriasis. The ratio of these two agents controls cellular replication. In psoriasis, cGMP levels are high in relation to cAMP levels. Silymarin works to lower cGMP levels while raising cAMP levels.

Summary

Silymarin, the flavonoid complex of *S. marianum*, is a potent liver-protecting substance useful in all types of liver disease and in psoriasis.

Dosage

The standard dose of *S. marianum* is based on its silymarin content (70–210 mg three times a day) which is why standardized extracts are preferred. Alcohol-based extracts are virtually always contraindicated due to the need to administer relatively high amounts of alcohol to obtain an adequate dose of silymarin.

Toxicology

Silymarin preparations are widely used medications in Europe, where a considerable body of evidence points to very low toxicity.[33] When used at high doses for short periods of time, silymarin given by various routes to mice, rats, rabbits, and dogs has shown no toxic effects. Studies in rats receiving silymarin for protracted periods have also demonstrated a complete lack of toxicity.

As silymarin possesses choleretic activity, it may produce a looser stool as a result of increased bile flow and secretion. If higher doses are used, it may be appropriate to use bile-sequestering fiber compounds (e.g., guar gum, pectin, psyllium, or oat bran) to prevent mucosal irritation and loose stools. Because of silymarin's lack of toxicity, long-term use is feasible when necessary.

References

1. Wagner H: Antihepatotoxic flavonoids. In: Plant Flavonoids in Biology and Medicine: Biochemical, Pharmacological, and Structure-Activity relationships. Edited by Cody V, Middleton E and Harbourne JB. Alan R Liss, Inc, New York, NY, 1986. pp545-58
2. Adzet T: Polyphenolic compounds with biological and pharmacological activity. Herbs Spices Medicinal Plants 1:167-84, 1986
3. Hikino H, Kiso Y, Wagner H, and Fiebig: Antihepatotoxic actions of flavanolignans from Silybum marianum fruits. Planta Medica 50:248-50, 1984

4. Wagner H: Plant constituents with antihepatotoxic activity. In: Natural Products as Medicinal Agents. Beal JL and Reinhard E (eds). Hippokrates-Verlag, Stuttgart, 1981
5. Vogel G, Tuchweber B, Trost W, and Mengs U: Protection against Amanita phalloides intoxication in beagles. Toxicol Appl Pharm 73:355-62, 1984
6. Desplaces A, Choppin J, Vogel G, and Trost W: The effects of silymarin on experimental phalloidin poisoning. Arzneim-Forsch 25:89-96, 1975
7. Vogel G, Trost W, Braatz R, et al: Studies on pharmacodynamics, site and mechanism of action of silymarin, the antihepatotoxic principle from Silybum marianum (L.) Gaert. Arzneim-Forsch 25:179-85, 1975
8. Zvenigorodskaia, LA and Speranskaia, I: Hepatoprotective preparations in the treatment of circulatory failure. Sov Med 3:67-71, 1988
9. Sarre H: Experience in the treatment of chronic hepatopathies with silymarin. Arzneim-Forsch 21:1209-12, 1971
10. Grieve M: A Modern Herbal, volume 1. Dover Publications, New York, NY, 1971. pp385-6
11. Sonnenbichler J, Goldberg M, Hane L, et al: Stimulatory effect of silibinin on the DNA synthesis in partially hepatectomized rat livers: non-response in hepatoma and other malignant cell lines. Biochem Pharm 35:538-41, 1986
12. Fiebrich F and Koch H: Silymarin, an inhibitor of lipoxygenase. Experentia 35:148-50, 1979
13. Fiebrich F and Koch H: Silymarin, an inhibitor of prostaglandin synthetase. Experentia 35:150-2, 1979
14. Sonnenbichler J and Zetl I: Biochemical effects of the flavanolignane silibinin on RNA, Protein and DNA synthesis in rat livers. In: Plant Flavonoids in Biology and Medicine: Biochemical, Pharmacological, and Structure-Activity relationships. Edited by Cody V, Middleton E and Harbourne JB. Alan R Liss, Inc, New York, NY, 1986. pp319-31
15. Schopen RD, Lange OK, Panne C, and Kirnberger EJ: Searching for a new therapeutic principle. Experience with hepatic therapeutic agent legalon. Med Welt 20:888-93, 1969
16. Schopen RD and Lange OK: Therapy of hepatoses. Therapeutic use of silymarin. Med Welt 21:691-8, 1970
17. Sarre H: Experience in the treatment of chronic hepatopathies with silymarin. Arzneim-Forsch 21:1209-12, 1971
18. Canini F, Bartolucci, Cristallini E, et al: Use of silymarin in the treatment of alcoholic hepatic steatosis. Clin Ter 114:307-14, 1985
19. Salmi HA and Sarna S: Effect of silymarin on chemical, functional, and morphological alteration of the liver. A double-blind controlled study. Scand J Gastroenterol 17:417-21, 1982
20. Scheiber V and Wohlzogen FX: Analysis of a certain type of 2 X 3 tables, exemplified by biopsy findings in a controlled clinical trial. Int J Clin Pharm 16:533-5, 1978
21. Boari C, Montanari M, Galleti GP, et al: Occupational toxic liver diseases. Therapeutic effects of silymarin. Min Med 72:2679-88
22. Grossi F and Viola F: Protettori di membrana e silimarina nella terapia epatologica. Cl Terap 96:11-23, 1981
23. Maneschi M, Tiberio C and Cittadini E: Impegno metabolico dell'epatocita in gravidanza: profilassi e terapia con un farmaco stabilizzante di membrana. Cl Terap 97:625-30, 1981
24. Bulfoni A and Gobbato F: Evaluation of the therapeutic activity of silymarine in alcoholic hepatology. Gazz Med Ital 138:597-608, 1979
25. Cavalieri S: A controlled clinical trial of Legalon in 40 patients. Gazz Med Ital 133:628-35
26. Saba P, Galeone GF, Salvadorini F, Guarguaglini M, and Troyer C: Therapeutic effects of silymarin in chronic liver diseases due to psychodrugs. Gazz Med Ital 135:236-51, 1976
27. De Martis M, Fontana M, Sebastiani F, and Parenzi A: La silymaina, farmaco membranotropo: ossevazioni cliniche e sperimentali. Cl Terap 81:333-62, 1977
28. Kock HP, Bachner J and Loffler E: Silymarin: Potent inhibitor of cyclic AMP phosphodiesterase. Meth Find Exptl Clin Pharm 7:409-13, 1985
29. Valenzuela A, Barria T, Guerra, and Garrido A: Inhibitory effect of the flavonoid silymarin on the erythrocyte hemolysis induced by phenylhydrazine. Biochem Biophys Res Comm 126:712-8, 1985
30. Flemming K: Effect of silymarin on X-radiated mice. Arzneim-Forsch 21:1373-5
31. Zoltan OT and Gyori I: Studies on the brain edema of the rat induced by triethyltinsulfate. Part 7: The therapeutic effect of silymarin, theophylline, and mannitol in the conditioned reflex test. Arzneim-Forsch 20:1248-9, 1970
32. Weber G and Galle K: The liver, a therapeutic target in dermatoses. Med Welt 34:108-11, 1983
33. Reynolds JE (ed): Martindale: The Extra Pharmacopoeia. Pharmaceutical Press, London, 1982. p1753
34. Valenzuela A, Lagos C, Schmidt K, and Videla LA: Silymarin protection against hepatic lipid peroxidation induced by acute ethanol intoxication in the rat. Biochem Pharm 34:2209-12, 1985
35. Seeger R: The effect of silymarin on osmotic resistance of erythrocytes. Arzneim-Forsch 21:1599-1605

9

Dandelion
(TARAXACUM OFFICINALE)

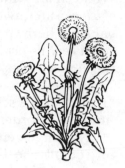

Key uses of dandelion root:

- Liver disorders
- Water retention
- Obesity

General description

The dandelion, familiar to almost everyone, is a perennial plant with an almost worldwide distribution. The spatula-shaped dentate leaves grow in a rosette formation from the milky taproot that also sends up one or more naked flower stems. The yellow flower is succeeded by the familiar puffball. The root is the portion of the plant that is used most extensively, although the leaves may have a greater diuretic effect.

Chemical composition

The dandelion offers greater nutritional value than many other vegetables. It is particularly high in vitamins and minerals, protein, choline, inulin, and pectins. Its carotenoid content is extremely high; it has a higher vitamin A content than carrots (dandelion has 14,000 IU of vitamin A per 100 g compared to 11,000 IU for carrots). Dandelion should be thought of as an extremely nutritious food and a rich source of medicinal compounds that have a toning effect on the body.[1,2]

History and folk use

While many individuals consider the common dandelion (*Taraxacum officinale*) an unwanted weed, herbalists all over the world have revered this valuable herb. Its common name, dandelion, is a corruption of the French word *dent-de-lion*, meaning "tooth-of-the-lion." Its common name describes the herb's leaves, which have several large, pointed teeth. Its scientific name, *Taraxacum*, is from the Greek *taraxos* (meaning "disorder") and *akos* (meaning "remedy"). Its scientific name alludes to dandelion's ability to correct a multitude of disorders.

Although generally regarded as a liver remedy, dandelion has a long history of folk use throughout the world. In Europe, dandelion was used in the treatment of fevers, boils, eye problems, diarrhea, fluid retention, liver congestion, heartburn, and various skin problems. In China, dandelion has been used to treat breast problems (cancer, inflammation, lack of milk flow, etc.), liver diseases, appendicitis, and digestive ailments. Dandelion's use in India, Russia, and other parts of the world revolved primarily around its action on the liver.[1,2]

Pharmacology

Liver effects

Dandelion is regarded as one of the finest liver remedies, as both food and medicine. Studies in humans and laboratory animals have shown that dandelion enhances the flow of bile, improving such conditions as liver congestion, bile duct inflammation, hepatitis, gallstones, and jaundice.[3,4] Dandelion's action on increasing bile flow is twofold: it has a direct effect on the liver, causing an increase in bile production and flow to the gallbladder (a choleretic effect), and a direct effect on the gallbladder, causing contraction and release of stored bile (a cholagogue effect). Dandelion's positive effect on such a wide variety of conditions is probably closely related to its ability to improve liver function.

Weight-loss aid and diuretic

Dandelion has been used historically as a weight-loss aid in the treatment of obesity, a fact that prompted researchers to investigate dandelion's effect on the body weight of experimental animals. When these animals were administered the fluid extract of dandelion for 1 month, they lost as much as 30% of their initial weights.[5] Much of the weight loss appeared to be a result of significant diuretic activity. The liver improving action, diuretic activity, and mild laxative effect of dandelion make it highly valued as a weight-loss aid.

Summary

Dandelion is a rich source of nutrients and other compounds that may improve liver functions, promote weight loss, and stimulate diuretic activity.

Dosage

As a general tonic and mild lipotropic (three times a day):

- Dried root (or as tea)—4 g
- Tincture—alcohol-based tinctures of dandelion are not recommended because of the extremely high dosage required
- Fluid extract (1:1)—4–8 ml (1–2 tsp)
- Powdered solid extract (4:1)—250–500 mg

References

1. Leung AY: Encyclopedia of Common Natural Ingredients Used in Food, Drugs and Cosmetics. John Wiley & Sons, New York, NY 1980
2. Duke JA: Handbook of Medicinal Herbs. CRC Press, Boca Raton, FL 1985
3. Mowrey DB: The Scientific Validation of Herbal Medicine. Cormorant Books, Lehi, UT 1986
4. Faber K: The dandelion - Taraxacum officinale Weber. Pharmazie 13:423-35, 1958
5. Racz-Kotilla E, Racz G and Solomon A: The action of Taraxacum officinale extracts on the body weight and diuresis of laboratory animals. Planta Medica 26:212-7, 1974

SECTION IV

Herbs for infections and immune-system enhancement

Many herbs have significant antibiotic activity against bacteria, viruses, fungi, and other microorganisms. However, herbs are much more than natural antibiotics. Modern scientific research is upholding what herbal practitioners have known for thousands of years—that many herbs work with the body's immune system to prevent as well as to treat infections. This section discusses four of the most highly respected and widely used herbal immune-system enhancers—goldenseal, echinacea, European mistletoe, and LaPacho.

10

Goldenseal

(HYDRASTIS CANADENSIS)

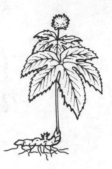

Key uses of goldenseal:

- Parasitic infections of the gastrointestinal tract
- Infections of mucous membranes
- Inflammation of the gallbladder
- Cirrhosis of the liver

General description

The plants *Hydrastis canadensis* (goldenseal), *Berberis vulgaris* (barberry), and *Mahonia aquifolium* (Oregon grape) share similar indications and effects because of their high content of berberis alkaloids. The chief berberis alkaloid, berberine, has been extensively studied in both experimental and clinical settings. This text gives the general description, history and folk use, chemical composition, and specific clinical indications for each plant. The pharmacology of the three plants is discussed primarily in terms of the activity of berberine.

Hydrastis Canadensis

Goldenseal is native to eastern North America and cultivated in Oregon and Washington. It is a perennial herb with a knotty yellow rhizome from which arises a single leaf and an erect, hairy stem. In early spring, it bears two five- to nine-lobed rounded leaves near the top, which are terminated by a single greenish-white flower. The parts used are the dried rhizome and the roots.[1,2]

Berberis Vulgaris

The common barberry is a deciduous spiny shrub that may reach 5 m in height. Native to Europe, it has been naturalized in eastern North America. The bark of the stem and the root are used.[1,2]

Mahonia Aquifolium

The Oregon grape is an evergreen spineless shrub, 1–2 m in height. It is native to the Rocky Mountains from British Columbia to California. Parts used are the rhizome and the roots.[1,2]

Chemical composition

Hydrastis Canadensis

Alkaloids isolated from hydrastis include: hydrastine (1.5–4.0%), berberine (0.5–6.0%), berberastine (2.0–3.0%), canadine, candaline, hydrastinine, and other related alkaloids. Other constituents include meconin, chlorogenic acid, phytosterins, and resins.[1,2]

Berberis Vulgaris

Barberry contains several alkaloids in its roots: jatrorrhizine, berberine, berberubine, berbamine, bervulcine, palmatine, columbamine, and oxyacanthine. It also contains chelidonic, citric, malic, and tartaric acids.[1,2]

Mahonia Aquifolium

Oregon grape contains the alkaloids berbamine, berberine, canadine, corypalmine, hydrastine, isocorydine, mahonine, and oxyacanthine. Resins and tannins have also been reported.[1,2]

History and folk use

Hydrastis Canadensis

Native to North America, goldenseal was used extensively by Native Americans as an herbal medication and clothing dye. Its medicinal use centered around its ability to soothe the mucous membranes that line the respiratory, digestive, and genitourinary tracts in inflammatory conditions induced by allergy or infection. The Cherokee and other Indian tribes also used goldenseal in disorders of the eye and skin.[1,2]

Berberis Vulgaris

This plant is native to most of Europe, and very similar species are found in North Africa and Asia. Barberry's historical use is as an antidiarrheal agent, bitter tonic, reducer of fever, and antihemorrhagic.[1,2]

Mahonia Aquifolium

The historical use and folk use of Oregon grape is similar to that of hydrastis. In addition, Oregon grape was used in the treatment of chronic skin conditions such as acne, psoriasis, and eczema.[1,2]

Pharmacology

The medicinal value of goldenseal, barberry, and Oregon grape is thought to result from their high content of isoquinoline alkaloids, of which berberine has been the most widely studied. Berberine has demonstrated antibiotic, immunostimulatory, anticonvulsant, sedative, hypotensive, uterotonic, cholerectic, and carminative activity. Berberine's pharmacological activities support the historical use of the berberine-containing herb.

Antibiotic activity

Perhaps the most celebrated of berberine's effects has been its antibiotic activity. Berberine exhibits a broad spectrum of antibiotic activity. Berberine has shown antimicrobial activity against bacteria, protozoa, and fungi, including *Stapyhlococcus* sp., *Streptococcus* sp., *Chlamydia* sp., *Corynebacterium diphtheria*, *Escherichia coli*, *Salmonella typhi*, *Vibrio cholerae*, *Diplococcus pneumonia*, *Pseudomonas* sp., *Shigella dysenteriae*, *Entamoeba histolytica*, *Trichomonas vaginalis*, *Neisseria gonorrhoeae* and *N. meningitidis*, *Treponema pallidum*, *Giardia lamblia*, *Leishmania donovani*, and *Candida albicans*.[1-9]

Its action against some of these pathogens (disease producing organisms) is actually stronger than that of antibiotics commonly used for diseases that these pathogens cause. Berberine-containing plants should be considered in infectious processes involving the above mentioned organisms. Berberine's action in inhibiting *Candida*, as well as pathogenic bacteria, prevents the overgrowth of yeast that is a common side effect of antibiotic use.

Anti-infective activity

Investigators decided to investigate berberine's ability to inhibit the adherence of group A streptococci to host cells since the therapeutic effect of berberine appeared to be greater than its direct antibiotic effects.[30] Recent studies have shown that some antimicrobial agents can block the adherence of microorganisms to host cells at doses much lower than those needed to kill cells or to inhibit cell growth.

Berberine is able to inhibit the adhesion of streptococci to host cells by several modes of action. First, berberine causes streptococci to lose lipoteichoic acid (LTA). LTA is the major substance responsible for the adhesion of the bacteria to host tissues. Another important action of berberine is preventing the adhesion of fibronectin to the streptococci as well as eluting (washing out) already bound fibronectin.

The significance of the results of this study are quite profound, raising many questions and forcing both researchers and practitioners to look at the treatment of bacterial infections in a new light. Is it better to utilize a substance with bactericidal or bacteriostatic actions over a substance that prevents the adherence of bacteria to host cells? Is the true value of botanicals that have anti-infective actions a multifactored effect on all aspects of infections, from immune stimulation to antimicrobial and antiadherence actions?

Simply stated, the results of the study indicate that berberine interferes with infections due to group A streptococci, not only by inhibiting streptococcal growth but also by blocking the adherence of these organisms to host cells. The study implies that berberine-containing plants may be ideal in the treatment of "strep throat," a condition American naturopathic physicians have traditionally healed with goldenseal. Berberine's action in inhibiting *Candida albicans* prevents the overgrowth of yeast that is a common side effect of antibiotic use.

Historically, berberine-containing plants have been used as febrifuges (fever-reducing agents). Berberine produced an antipyretic effect three times as potent as aspirin in a fever model in rats.[29]

Immunostimulatory activity

Berberine has been shown to increase the blood supply to the spleen.[10] This improved blood supply may promote optimal activity of the spleen, an organ responsible for filtering the blood and releasing compounds that potentiate immune function. Berberine has also been shown to activate macrophages,[11] cells responsible for engulfing and destroying bacteria, viruses, tumor cells, and other particulate matter.

Therapeutic use in treating infections

The broad antimicrobial effects of berberine, combined with its anti-infective and immune-stimulating actions, supports the historical use of berberine-containing plants in infections of the mucous membranes—i.e., the linings of the oral cavity, throat, sinuses, bronchi, genitourinary tract, and gastrointestinal tract.

Berberine has shown significant success in the treatment of acute diarrhea in several clinical studies. It has been found effective against diarrheas caused by *E. coli* (traveler's diarrhea), *Shigella dysenteriae* (shigellosis), *Salmonella* sp. (food poisoning), *B. Klebsiella*, *Giardia lamblia* (giardiasis), and *Vibrio cholerae* (cholera).[6,12-16] Studies in hamsters and rats have shown that berberine also has significant activity against *Entamoeba histolytica*, the causative organism of amebiasis.

In addition to its direct antimicrobial activity, experimental results indicate that berberine-containing plants are particularly appropriate in diarrheas caused by enterotoxins (e.g., *Vibrio cholerae* and *E. coli*).[18-21] It thus appears that berberine is effective in treating the majority of common gastrointestinal infections.

For those planning to travel to a developing country or an area that has poor water quality or sanitation, the prophylactic use of berberine-containing herbs during the visit, 1 week prior to leaving and 1 week following return may be useful.

Therapeutic use for trachoma

Cultures throughout the world have used water extracts of berberine-containing plants to treat a variety of eye complaints, including infectious processes. In recent times, berberine has shown remarkable effect in the treatment of trachoma,[22,23] an infectious eye disease caused by the organism *Chlamydia trachomatis* and a major cause of blindness and impaired vision in developing countries. Trachoma affects approximately 500 million people worldwide and results in blindness in 2 million.

The drug sulphacetamide is currently the most widely used antitrachoma drug. In clinical trials comparing berberine (0.2%) and sulphacetamide (20.0% solution), sulphacetamide showed the best improvement (marked by a decrease in conjunctival discharge, edema, and papillary reactions).[22,23] However, the conjunctival scrapings of all patients receiving sulphacetamide were still positive for *C. trachomatis*. These patients had a high rate of recurrence of the symptoms. In contrast, patients treated with the berberine solution showed very mild ocular symptoms, which disappeared more gradually, but their conjunctival scrapings were always negative for *C. trachomatis*. These patients did not suffer relapse even 1 year after treatment, which suggests that berberine is probably curative for trachoma.

Berberine's effect is believed to be due to stimulation of some host defense mechanism rather than a direct action on the organism. Because the berberine concentration used in these studies was 100 times less than the concentration of sulphacetamide, and berberine is much less expensive than sulphacetamine, berberine may be more cost effective than other treatments for trachoma. Berberine (0.2% solution) is appropriate therapy for many types of conjunctivitis.

Therapeutic use for cholecystitis and cirrhosis of the liver

Berberine has been shown in several clinical studies to stimulate the secretion of bile (cholerectic effect) and bilirubin.[24,25] Turova et al. examined the effect of berberine on 225 patients who suffered chronic cholecystitis (inflammation of the gallbladder). Oral doses of 5–20 mg of berberine three times a day before meals caused, over a period of 24–48 hr, disappearance of clinical symptoms, a decrease in bilirubin level, and an increase in the bile volume of the gallbladder. Berberine also has been shown to correct metabolic abnormalities in patients who suffer liver cirrhosis.[26-28]

Summary

No detailed clinical studies have differentiated which berberine-containing herb to use for specific conditions. The following indications are offered only as a guideline, based on experimental studies and historical use:

Hydrastis canadensis indications:
  Infective, congestive, and inflammatory states of the mucous membranes, digestive disorders, gastritis, peptic ulcers, colitis, anorexia, painful menstruation.
Berberis vulgaris indications:
  Gallbladder disease, including gallstones, and as a less expensive form of berberine in the treatment of the conditions listed for *Hydrastis*.
Mahonia aquifolium indications:
  Chronic skin diseases and the conditions listed for *Hydrastis*.

Dosage

Three times a day dosages:

- Dried root or as infusion (tea)—2–4 g
- Tincture (1:5)—6–12 ml (1½–3 tsp)
- Fluid extract (1:1)—1–2 ml (¼–½ tsp)
- Solid (powdered dry) extract (4:1 or 8–12% alkaloid content)—250–500 mg

Toxicology

Berberine and berberine-containing plants are generally nontoxic at the recommended dosages. However, berberine-containing plants are not recommended for use during pregnancy, and high dosages may interfere with the metabolism of B vitamins.

References

1. Duke JA: Handbook of Medicinal Herbs. CRC Press, Boca Raton, Fl 1985. pp78, 238-9, 287-8
2. Leung AY: Encyclopedia of Common Natural Ingredients Used in Food, Drugs, and Cosmetics. John Wiley & Sons, New York, NY 1980. pp52-3, 189-90
3. Hahn FE and Ciak J: Berberine. Antibiotics 3:577-88, 1976
4. Amin AH, Subbaiah TV and Abbasi KM: Berberine sulfate: Antimicrobial activity, bioassay, and mode of action. Can J Microbiol 15:1067-76, 1969
5. Johnson CC, Johnson G and Poe CF: Toxicity of alkaloids to certain bacteria. Acta Pharmacol Toxicol 8:71-8, 1952
6. Choudry VP, Sabir M and Bhide VN: Berberine in giardiasis. Ind Pediatr 9:143-6, 1972
7. Subbaiah TV and Amin AH: Effect of berberine sulfate on Entamoeba histolytica. Nature 215:527-8, 1967
8. Ghosh AK: Effect of berberine chloride on Leishmania donovani. Ind J Med Res 78:407-16, 1983
9. Majahan VM, Sharma A and Rattan A: Antimycotic activity of berberine sulphate: An alkaloid from an Indian medicinal herb. Sabouraudia 20:79-81, 1982
10. Sabir M and Bhide N: Study of some pharmacologic actions of berberine. Ind J Physiol Pharm 15:111-32, 1971
11. Kumazawa Y, Itagaki A, Fukumoto M, et al: Activation of peritoneal macrophages by berberine alkaloids in terms of induction of cytostatic activity. Int J Immunopharmacol 6:587-92, 1984
12. Gupta S: Use of berberine in the treatment of giardiasis. Am J Dis Child 129:866, 1975
13. Bhakat MP, Nandi N, Pal HK and Khan BS: Therapeutic trial of Berberine sulphate in non-specific gastroenteritis. Ind Med J 68:19-23, 1974
14. Kamat SA: Clinical trial with berberine hydrochloride for the control of diarrhoea in acute gastroenteritis. J Assoc Physicians India 15:525-9, 1967
15. Desai AB, Shah KM and Shah DM: Berberine in the treatment of diarrhoea. Ind Pediatr 8:462-5, 1971
16. Sharma R, Joshi CK and Goyal RK: Berberine tannate in acute diarrhea. Ind Pediatr 7:496-501, 1970
17. Khin-Maung-U, Myo-Khin, Nyunt-Wai, et al: Clinical trial of berberine in acute watery diarrhoea. Br Med J 291:1601-5, 1985
18. Sack RB and Froehlich JL: Berberine inhibits intestinal secretory response of vibrio cholerae toxins and Escherichia coli enterotoxins. Infect Immun 35:471-5, 1982
19. Tai YH, Feser JF, Mernane WG and Desjeux JF: Antisecretory effects of berberine in rat ileum. Am J Physiol 241:G253-8, 1981

20. Swabb EA, Tai YH and Jordan L: Reversal of cholera toxin-induced secretion in rat ileum by luminal berberine. Am J Physiol 241:G248-52, 1981
21. Akhter MH, Sabir M and Bhide NK: Possible mechanism of antidiarrhoeal effect of berberine. Ind J Med Res 70:233-41, 1979
22. Babbar OP, Chatwal VK, Ray IB and Mehra MK: Effect of berberine chloride eye drops on clinically positive trachoma patients. Ind J Med Res 76(Suppl):83-8, 1982
23. Mohan M, Pant CR, Angra SK and Mahajan VM: Berberine in trachoma. Ind J Opthalmol 30:69-75, 1982
24. Preininger V: The pharmacology and toxicology of the papaveraceae alkaloids. Alkaloids 15:207-51, 1975
25. Chan MY: The effect of berberine on bilirubin excretion in the rat. Comp Med East West 5:161-8, 1977
26. Watanabe A, Obata T and Nagashima H: Berberine therapy of hypertyraminemia in patients with liver cirrhosis. Acta Med Okayama 36:277-81, 1982
27. Kuwano S and Yamauchi K: Effect of berberine on tyrosinase decarboxylase activity of Streptococcus faecalis. Chem Pharm Bull 8:491-6, 1960
28. Kuwano S and Yamauchi K: Effect of berberine with pyridoxal phosphate in the tryptophanase system of Escherichia coli. Chem Pharm Bull 8:497-503, 1960
29. Sabir M, Akhter MH and Bhide NK: Further studies on pharmacology of berberine. Ind J Physiol Pharmacol 22:9-23, 1978
30. Sun D, Courtney HS and Beachey EH: Berberine sulfate blocks adherence of Streptococcus pyogenes to epithelial cells, fibronectin, and hexadecane. Antimicrobial Agents and Chemotherapy 32:1370-4, 1988

11

Echinacea

(ECHINACEA ANGUSTIFOLIA AND ENCHINACEA PURPUREA)

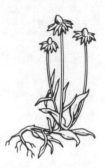

Key uses of echinacea root:

- Viral infections
- Impaired immune function
- Wound healing

General description

Echinacea is a perennial herb native to the midwestern region of North America, from Saskatchewan to Texas. It grows 2–3 ft high; has thick, hairy leaves, 3–8 in. long; and produces a characteristic large, pale purple flower. The dried root is typically used for its medicinal value.

Chemical composition

The following compounds have been isolated from echinacea: inulin, glucose, fructose, betaine, echinacin, echinacoside, trihydroxyphenyl propionic acid, resins, essential oils, and fatty acids.[1]

History and folk use

Echinacea was introduced into American medicine in 1885 by Dr. H. C. F. Meyer, who recommended it as a "blood purifier."[2] The Indian tribes of Nebraska used it as an antiseptic and analgesic, and the Sioux used it as a snakebite remedy. Eclectic practitioners used it externally as a local antiseptic, stimulant, deodorant, and anesthetic, and internally to treat "bad blood"—i.e., to correct "fluid depravation with tendency to sepsis and malignancy."[3]

Pharmacology

Wound healing and anti-inflammatory properties

Echinacin, a polysaccharide component of echinacea, has been shown to promote wound healing in experimental studies,[2] apparently due to its ability to maintain the structure and integrity of the collagen matrix in connective tissue and ground substance. Echinacea also has some cortisonelike properties.[4,5]

Echinacea has quite a reputation among naturopathic physicians and Native American healers for the treatment of snakebites. Snake venom contains hyaluronidase, "the spreading factor," which breaks down ground substance and allows the venom to penetrate into the bloodstream. Echinacea contains compounds that have demonstrated potent inhibition of hyaluronidase. This characteristic might account for much of echinacea's reputed effect as a snakebite venom.

Immune-enhancing properties

Echinacea's major component, inulin, is an activator of the alternative complement pathway, which is responsible for increasing host defense mechanisms like the neutralization of viruses, the destruction of bacteria, and an increased movement of white blood cells (neutrophils, monocytes, eosinophils, and lymphocytes) to areas of infection.

Echinacea has also shown to increase properdin levels.[6] This compound is the body's natural activator of the alternative complement pathway. This double activation of complement may be responsible for much of echinacea's antibiotic and anticancer effects.

Further studies have shown that echinacea has other components with profound immunostimulatory effects.[6-8,13] The components responsible for these effects are primarily polysaccharides that are able to bind to carbohydrate receptors on the cell surface of T-lymphocytes and other white blood cells. This binding results in nonspecific T-cell activation, including transformation, increased production of interferon, and secretion of lymphokines. The resultant effect is enhanced T-cell mitogenesis (reproduction), macrophage phagocytosis (the engulfment and destruction of bacteria or viruses), antibody binding, natural killer cell activity, and increased levels of circulating neutrophils (white blood cells primarily responsible for defense against bacteria). Echinacea's caffeinic acid content may also exert some mild antibacterial action.

Antiviral properties

Root extracts of echinacea have been shown to possess interferon-like properties.[9] Interferon is a compound produced in the body that stimulates the synthesis of proteins that block viral infection. In addition, echinacea has demonstrated specific antiviral activity against influenza, herpes, and vesicular stomatitis viruses.[9]

Echinacea's antiviral effects may also be due to inhibition of hyaluronidase. Many organisms secrete hyaluronidase, which increases ground substance permeability and allows the organism to become more invasive.[10]

Anticancer activity

During experimental studies, (Z)-1,8-pentadecadiene, a lipid-soluble component of the root, has been shown to promote significant anticancer activity.[12]

Summary

Echinacea causes potent immunostimulatory activity via activation of the alternative complement pathway, activation of T-lymphocytes and other white blood cells, promotion of interferon production and secretion, antiviral activity, and its ability to decrease the infectivity of the organism. These effects make echinacea useful as a general enhancer of the immune system, especially during an infectious process.

Dosage

As a general immune stimulant during infection (three times a day doses):

- Dried root (or as tea)—1–2 g
- Tincture (1:5)—8–12 ml (2–3 tsp.)
- Fluid extract (1:1)—2–4 ml (0.5–1 tsp.)
- Solid (dry powdered) extract (6.5:1)—250–500 mg

Toxicology

Echinacea is regarded as an extremely safe herb with no reported toxicity.

References

1. Merck Index, 10th ed, p 3473, Merck & Co, 1983
2. Tyler V, Brady L and Robbers J: Pharmacognosy, 8th ed. Lea & Febiger, Philadelphia, Pa, 1981. pp480-1
3. Felter H: The Eclectic Materia Medica, Pharmacology and Therapeutics. Eclectic Medical Publ, Portland, Or 1983. pp347-351
4. Koch F and Haase H: Eine Modifikation des spreading-testes im tierversuch, gleichzeitig ein beitrag zum wirkungsmechanismus von echinacin. Arzneim Forsch 2:464-7, 1952
5. Busing K: Hyaluronidasehemmung durch echinacin. Arzneim Forsch 2:467-9, 1952
6. Mose J: Effect of echinacin on phagocytosis and natural killer cells. Med Welt 34:1463-7, 1983
7. Wagner V, Proksch A, Riess-Maurer I, et al: Immunostimulating polysaccharides (heteroglycanes) of higher plants / preliminary communications. Arzneim Forsch 34:659-660, 1984
8. Vomel V: Influence of a non-specific immune stimulant on phagocytosis of erythrocytes and ink by the reticuloendothelial system of isolated perfused rat livers of different ages. Arzneim Forsch 34:691-5, 1984
9. Wacker A and Hilbig W: Virus-inhibition by echinacea purpurea. Planta Medica 33:89-102, 1978
10. Hopp E and Burn H: Ground substance in the nose in health and infection. Annals Oto Rhino Laryngol 65:480-9, 1956
11. Cizmarik J and Matle I: Examination of the chemical composition of propolis I. Isolation and identification of the 3,4, dihydroxycinnamic acid (caffeic acid) from propolis. Experentia 26:713,1970
12. Voaden D and Jacobson M: Tumor inhibitors. 3. Identification and synthesis of an oncolytic hydrocarbon from American coneflower roots. J Med Chem 15:619-23, 1972
13. Bauer VR, Jurcic K, Puhlmann J and Wagner H: Immunological in vivo and in vitro examinations of echinacea extracts. Arzneim Forsch 38:276-81, 1988

12

European mistletoe

(VISCUM ALBUM)

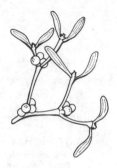

Key uses of European mistletoe:

- High blood pressure
- Cancer
- Impaired thymus gland activity
- Immune system enhancement

General description

Viscum album, or European mistletoe, is an evergreen, semiparasitic plant found on the branches of deciduous trees in Europe and northern Asia. The roots of the plant penetrate through the bark into the wood of the host tree. The green branches 40–60 cm long form pendent bushes with leaves that are opposite, leathery, yellow-green and narrowly obovate. Pale yellow or green inconspicuous flowers appear from March to May. The female flowers develop into sticky white berries that ripen from September to November.[1,2]

Mistletoe most commonly is seen on old apple, ash, and hawthorn trees. Traditionally, mistletoe from oak has been the most widely used, although it does not grow as well on oak as it does on the previously mentioned trees.[1,2]

Chemical composition

V. album contains a variety of pharmacologically active substances, including alkaloids, polysaccharides, phenylpropanes, lignans, lectins, and "viscotoxins."[3-10] Specific compounds found in mistletoe include a wide range of carbohydrates, including simple sugars as well as polysaccharides;[5] phenolic compounds such as flavonoids, caffeic acid, syringin, and eleutherosides;[6,10]

sterols, including beta-sitosterol, stigmasterol, and triterpenes; various amino acids and vasoactive amines, including tyramine, phenylethylamine, and histamine; and fatty acids such as linoleic, palmitic, and oleic acids.[2]

The alkaloids isolated from mistletoe appear to be related to those found in the host plant.[3,4] For example, mistletoe growing on solanaceae shrubs contain nicotine alkaloids like hyoscine, anabasine, and isopelletierine; cardiac glycosides have been found in mistletoe growing on *Nerium oleander;* strychnine has been found in mistletoe growing on *Strychnos* sp.; and caffeine has been found in mistletoe growing on coffee plants.

Because pharmacologically active compounds appear to be concentrated within the mistletoe, different host trees providing different chemical constituents could be used for different therapeutic action. In addition, the proteins and lectins are present only in aqueous (water) extracts, which indicates that therapeutic activity may differ from aqueous and alcohol/aqueous (tinctures) extracts. The alcohol/aqueous extracts would also demonstrate considerably less toxicity.

History and folk use

The Druids held mistletoe in great reverence. Dressed in white robes, the Druids would search for the sacred plant. When they discovered it, they would conduct a great ceremony in which a Druid would use a golden knife to separate the mistletoe from the oak. The Druids believed that the mistletoe protected them from all evil, and the oaks on which it was seen growing were to be respected because of the wonderful cures the priests were able to produce with the mistletoe.[1]

Mistletoe's use was recorded in the Middle East, Africa, India, and Japan. Mistletoe was mentioned as an anticancer drug by Pliny, Dioscorides, and Galen.[3]

In 1720, English physician Sir John Colbatch extolled the virtues of mistletoe in a pamphlet titled "The Treatment of Epilepsy by Mistletoe." For many years, mistletoe was used in the treatment of a variety of nervous system disorders, including convulsions, delirium, hysteria, neuralgia, and nervous debility.[1,3]

Probably due to toxicity, use of *Viscum album* appeared to fall into some disrepute shortly after Colbatch's work. For many years, it was used only in external preparations for the treatment of dermatitis. In 1906, a study that demonstrated mistletoe's hypotensive action in animals and humans was published. This appears to have restored the medical prestige of *V. album,* initially in France and eventually throughout Europe.[3]

Pharmacology

V. album exhibits diverse pharmacological actions. The herb and various extracts have demonstrated hypotensive, vasodilating, cardiac depressant, sedative, antispasmodic, immunostimulatory, and antineoplastic activities.

Cardiovascular effects

V. album has exhibited a variety of effects on components of the cardiovascular system.[3,11] Specifically, it has repeatedly demonstrated blood pressure lowering action in animal studies. The mechanism of action for this effect is still not entirely clear because no recent investigations exist. Mistletoe has been shown to affect blood pressure control centers in the brain.[11]

The blood pressure lowering activity may be dependent on the form in which the mistletoe is administered and on the host tree from which it was collected. Studies indicate aqueous extracts are more effective, and the highest hypotensive activity was demonstrated by a macerate of leaves of mistletoe parasitizing on willow and gathered in January.[11]

Nonprotein components of *V. album* (e.g., flavonoids, phenol carboxylic acids, phenylpropanes and lignans) were shown to cause blood pressure lowering action. Alcohol solutions (tinctures and fluid extracts) contained these components but not viscotoxins or lectins. However, aqueous extracts appear to be more effective.

In Europe, several mistletoe preparations for hypertension exist. In fact, in Britain alone there are more than 150 different mistletoe preparations on the market.[3] These preparations typically have small amounts of *Viscum* in combination with other botanicals thought to have hypotensive action (e.g., garlic, *Crataegus oxyacantha*, and *Tilia platyphyllos*).

Anticancer and immunostimulatory effects

Mistletoe preparations have been used clinically in Europe in the treatment of cancers since 1926, when a fermented product, Iscador, made from the crude juice of the pressed plant was introduced as a therapeutic agent for cancer. This work was carried out under the direction of Rudolph Steiner. Since that time, numerous studies have been performed on this preparation as well as other mistletoe preparations and components.[12-31]

It must be pointed out that Iscador is injected under the skin or into the blood. It is not known to what degree (if any) the effects noted for Iscador, as well as other preparations and compounds, are able to be achieved with oral administration.

Iscador and other fermented mistletoe preparations differ from nonfermented extracts in several ways that are thought to reduce toxicity and increase effectiveness.[12] Specifically, the major viscotoxin, ML I, is not found in Iscador.[13] Fermentation results in a rapid decrease of lectin concentration. It is thought that ML I is transformed to its A and B chains. These chains have important immunological properties.[14]

The pharmacological activity of Iscador has been shown to be due to the mistletoe components rather than to other constituents. Iscador does contain lactobacilli, which promote immune-enhancing activity. It has been clearly demonstrated that the lectins are the mistletoe components largely responsible for Iscador's activity because unfermented plant juice has demonstrated comparable activity to Iscador.[15,16]

Iscador is most effective when administered near the tumor (i.e., locally), although systemic administration has also yielded positive results. Upon local administration, an inflammatory process ensues that promotes white blood cell infiltration and a "walling off" of the tumor.

The nonspecific host defense factors stimulated by *V. album* include enhanced macrophage phagocytic and cytotoxic activity;[12,16] increased numbers of neutrophils; increased thymic weight and enhanced cortical thymocyte activity and proliferation;[17,19] enhanced natural killer cell activity;[12,18,20] and increased antibody-dependent, cell-mediated cytotoxicity.[12,18] Iscador's effects on these immunological parameters have been confirmed in patients who have cancer.[12,18]

Iscador's effect on stimulating the thymus gland has been demonstrated in several studies.[17,19] Its ability to stimulate the thymic cortex and accelerate the regeneration of hematopoietic cells following X-irradiation is much greater than anything else reported to date.[17] In addition, thymic lymphocytes became 29 times more responsive to concanavalin A as a result of Iscador administration.

It is interesting to note that purified mistletoe lectins, in general, are not as active in experimental studies as crude preparations.[21,22] Presumably there are a number of compounds in mistletoe that act synergistically. It has also been proposed that alkaloid components are responsible for the maintenance of lectin structure and activity.[5] During isolation and purification procedures, alkaloid linkages are cleaved from the lectins, resulting in a loss of specifity for target molecules. Unfermented preparations of *V. album* typically demonstrate a greater direct toxicity to tumor cells because of higher concentrations of the viscotoxin ML I.[14,23,24]

Essentially, *V. album* exhibits numerous immunostimulatory effects that indicate a therapeutic effect in human cancer. These effects have been confirmed against various tumors in mice.[4]

Early clinical investigations of mistletoe preparations (i.e., Iscador) were not very well documented. Due to the lack of acceptable scientifically controlled clinical trials, the use of Iscador as a cancer treatment in Europe has remained controversial. Recently, several clinical trials have been started that should provide greater information as to the effectiveness of Iscador. It has already been demonstrated that the use of Iscador in the postoperative treatment of lung, breast, colon, and cervical carcinomas is of benefit.[25-27]

Summary

Clearly, additional investigations on the pharmacology of *V. album* are needed. Specifically, science must determine if the same effects noted in animals and in patients receiving injections of mistletoe preparations can be attained by oral administration of such preparations.

In addition, greater clarification is needed to determine optimal mistletoe preparations. What host tree should be selected for which condition? What is the optimal harvesting time? In what form should *Viscum* be administered— crude herb, aqueous or alcohol extract, fermented or nonfermented?

Mistletoe is undoubtedly one of the most complex botanicals. Yet, after examining currently available data, it can be said with much confidence that the future medicinal use of *V. album* is quite promising.

Dosage

The standard dose of *V. album* based on the information given in the *British Herbal Pharmacopoeia* is as follows:

- Dried leaves—2–6 g (or by infusion), 3 x/day
- Tincture of 1:5 (45% alcohol)—1–3 ml, 3 x/day
- Fluid extract of 1:1 (25% alcohol)—0.5 ml, 3 x/day
- Dried aqueous extract (4:1)—100–250 mg, 3 x/day

Toxicology

V. album possesses significant toxicity. Historically, the berries have been regarded as being significantly more toxic than the leaves and stems, despite the fact that these latter parts contain similar toxic compounds. The reason the toxicity of the berries is considered greater probably derives from the fatal poisonings that have occurred after ingestion of the berries.

Lethal doses of *Viscum* lectins administered by various routes in mice produced two types of toxicity: a typical type characterized by death after 3–4 days of experiencing marasmus-like symptoms, and an atypical type characterized by immediate death caused by respiratory paralysis.[19]

The definitive toxicity of orally administered *V. album* or its extracts have not yet been determined. As stated earlier, alcohol based extracts contain virtually no *Viscum* proteins. This would imply that these types of preparations are significantly less toxic. However, it also would imply that they are less active because the pharmacology of mistletoe relates to its protein content (especially for its immune-enhancing activity).

It is interesting to note that the toxicity of Korean mistletoe, *V. a. coloratum,* appears to be less than that of European mistletoe.[30,31] This species has also demonstrated anticancer effects, but the effects appear to be due to alkaloids rather than to lectins.[5,30] In studies that compared Korean mistletoe extracts to European mistletoe extracts, as well as their alkaloid components, Korean mistletoe showed greater activity in inhibiting cancer cells. In addition, fresh Korean mistletoe extracts exhibited greater activity compared to fermented extracts.[5,30] In the future, Korean mistletoe may prove superior to European mistletoe.

References

1. Grieve M: A Modern Herbal. Dover Publications, New York, NY, 1971 pp547-8
2. Becker H: Botany of European Mistletoe (Viscum album L.). Oncology 43:suppl.1;2-7, 1986
3. Anderson LA and Phillippson JD: Mistletoe - the magic herb.
4. Khwaja TA, Dias CB and Pentecost S: Recent studies on the anticancer activities of mistletoe (Viscum album) and its alkaloids. Oncology 43:suppl.1;42-50, 1986
5. Jordan E and Wagner H: Structure and properties of polysaccharides from Viscum album (L.). Oncology 43:suppl.1;8-15, 1986
6. Wagner H, Jordan E and Feil B: Studies on the standardization of mistletoe preparations. Oncology 43:suppl.1;16-22, 1986
7. Franz H, Ziska P and Kindt A: Isolation and properties of three lectins from mistletoe (Viscum album L.). Biochem J 195:481-4, 1981
8. Olsnes S, Stirpe F, Sandvig K and Phil A: Isolation and characterisation of viscumin, a toxic lectin from Viscum album L. (mistletoe). J Biol Chem 257:13263-70, 1982
9. Petricic J and Kalogjera Z: Isolation of glucosides from mistletoe leaves (Viscum album L.). Acta Pharm Jugosl 30:163, 1980
10. Wagner H, Feil B, Kalogjera Z and Petricic J: Phenylpropanes and lignanes of Viscum album. Planta Medica 2:102, 1986
11. Petkov V: Plants with hypotensive, antiatheromatous and coronarodilatating action. Am J Chin Med 7:197-236, 1979
12. Hajto T: Immunomodulating effects of Iscador: a Viscum album preparation. Oncology 43:suppl.1;51-65, 1986
13. Jordan E and Wagner H: Detection and quantitative determination of lectins and viscotoxins in mistletoe preparations. Arzneim Forsch 36:428-33, 1986
14. Ribereau-Gayon G, Jung ML, Di Scala D and Beck JP: Comparison of the effects of fermented and unfermented mistletoe preparations on cultured tumor cells. ONcology 43:suppl.1;35-41, 1986
15. Bloksma N, Dijk HV, Korst P and Willers JM: Cellular and humoral adjuvant activity of a mistletoe extract. Immunobiol 156:309-19, 1979
16. Bloksma N, Schmiermann P, Reuver MD, Dijk HD and Willers J: Stimulation of humoral and cellular immunity by viscum preparations. Planta Medica 46:221-7, 1982

17. Rentea R, Lyon E and Hunter R: Biological properties of Iscador: a Viscum album preparation. Lab Invest 44:43-8, 1981
18. Hajto T and Lanzrein: Natural killer and antibody-dependent cell-mediated cytotoxicity activities and large granular lymphocyte frequencies in Viscum album-treated breast cancer patients. Oncology 43:93-7, 1986
19. Nienhaus J, Stoll M and Vester F: Thymus stimulation and cancer prophylaxis by Viscum proteins. Experentia 26:523-5, 1970
20. Hamprecht K, Handretinger R, Voetsch W and Anderer FA: Mediation of human NK-activity by components in extracts of Viscum album. Int J Immunopharm 9:199-209, 1987
21. Evans MR and Preece AW: Viscum album - a possible treatment for cancer? Bristol Med Chir J 88:17-20, 1973
22. Klamerth O, Vester F and Kellner G: Inhibitory effects of a protein complex from Viscum album on fibroblasts and HeLa cells. Z Physiol Chem 349:863-4, 1968
23. Hulsen H, Doser C and Mechelke F: Differences in the in vitro effectiveness of preparations produced from mistletoes of various host trees. Arzneim Forsch 36:433-6, 1986
24. Hulsen H and Mechelke F: THe influence of a mistletoe preparation on suspension cell cultures of human leukemia and human myeloma cells. Arzneim Forsch 32:1126-7, 1982
25. Leroi R: Nachbehandling des operierten mammakarzinoms mit Viscum allbum. Helv Chir Acta 44:403-14, 1977
26. Leroi R: Neuere resultate aus dem gebeit del malignombehandlung mit Viscum album. Erfahrungsheilkunde 25:41-54, 1977
27. Salzer G and Havelec L: Rezidivprophyl bei operierten bronchuskarzinoompatiienten mit mistelpraparat Iscador. Onkologie 1:264-7, 1978
28. Duke JA: Handbook of Medicinal Herbs. CRC Press, Boca Raton, FL, 1986, pp512-3
29. British Herbal Medicine Association, Scientific Committee: British Herbal Pharmacopoeia. British Herbal Medicine Association, Cowling, England, 1983, pp235-6
30. Khwaja TA, Varven JC, Pentecost S and Pande H: Isolation of biologically active alkaloids from Korean mistletoe Viscum album, coloratum. Experentia 36:599-600, 1980
31. Manjikian S, Pentecost S and Khwaja TA: Isolation of cytotoxic proteins form Viscum album, coloratum. Proc Am Ass Cancer Res 27:266, 1986

13

LaPacho

(TABEBUIA AVELLANEDAE)

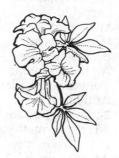

Key uses of LaPacho:

- Infections
- Cancer
- *Candida albicans*

General description

Although there are about 100 *Tabebuia* species native to tropical America, *Tabebuia avellanedae* or *T. ipe* is regarded as the true "LaPacho." This tree, native to Brazil, can rise to a height of 125 ft and has rose- to violet-colored flowers that bloom in profusion just before the new leaves appear. The bark is the portion of the tree that is used medicinally.

Chemical composition

Many of the studies and chemical analyses on *Tabebuia* sp. have been done on the heartwood, although the bark is the product available in the marketplace and the part used as a folk remedy. The major components of *T. avellanedae* are 16 quinones (mostly with C_{15} skeleton) containing both naphthoquinones (7, C_{10}–C_5) and anthraquinones (9, C_{14}–C_1); it is considered very rare to have both these groups of quinones occurring in the same plant. The lapachol content is usually 2–7%. The quinones are listed in Table 1. Other compounds found in the heartwood are lapachenole, quercetin, and *o*- and *p*-hydroxybenzoic acids.[2]

A recent analysis of 12 products found in the Canadian marketplace showed that one contained trace amounts of lapachol and the other 11 contained none. This suggests that many of the products on the market are not

Table 1 Quinones in *T. avellanedae*

Naphthoquinones
Lapachol
Menaquinone-l
Deoxylapachol
Beta-lapachone
Alpha-lapachone
Dehydro-alpha-lapachone
Anthraquinones
2-Methylanthraquinone
2-Hydroxymethylanthraquinone
2-Acetoxymethylanthraquinone
Anthraquinone-2-aldehyde
1-Hydroxyanthraquinone
1-Methoxyanthraquinone
2-Hydroxy-3-methylquinone
Tabebuin (a newly discovered compound)

truly *Tabebuia* sp., that the wrong part of the plant is being marketed, or that processing and transportation have damaged the product. This might explain the variation in results that practitioners have experienced. Standardizing LaPacho products for lapachol or naphthoquinone content would obviously solve this problem.

History and folk use

The Indians of Brazil also refer to the LaPacho tree as Pau D'Arco or Ipe Roxo. They have used the inner bark of the tree for centuries as a folk remedy for a wide variety of afflictions, including boils; chlorosis; colitis; diarrhea; dysentery; bedwetting; fever; sore throat; snakebite; syphilis; wounds; cancer of the esophagus, head, intestine, lung, prostate, and tongue; ulcers, respiratory problems; arthritis; cystitis; constipation; prostatitis; poor circulation; and constipation.[4-7]

Pharmacology

During the past century, LaPacho has come under scientific scrutiny. The first active constituent to be studied was lapachol, which was isolated by Paterno (in 1882) and whose structure was determined by Hooker in 1896. In

1927, Fieser synthesized lapachol. It has since been studied by numerous scientists.

It is interesting to note that many of the scientific studies show significantly better results with the whole extract and diminishing effectiveness as the extracts are refined or individual chemicals are tested.[8]

Antibacterial activity

In 1956, a research team at the Universidade do Recife in Brazil isolated lapachol from the *T. avellanedae* tree. De Lima and his colleagues reported that it exhibited antimicrobial activity against gram-positive and acid-fast bacteria and showed strong activity against *Brucella* sp.[9]

It is important to note that de Lima and his team found that with progressive purification the antimicrobial activity of the extract decreased. This led to the conclusion that there was more than one active substance present in the original extract.

Later that year the team published a paper proclaiming a new antibiotic substance from *T. avellanedae* that demonstrated "strong anti-*Brucella* activity and fungistatic behavior."[10] De Lima's team eventually found that, along with lapachol, the extract of the LaPacho tree contains alpha-lapachone, beta-lapachone, and a newly discovered quinone, which they named xyloidone.

In 1967, at the University of Aberdeen, the team of Burnett and Thomson discovered the presence of seven naphthoquinones, nine anthraquinones, lapachenole, quercetin, and *o*- and *p*-hydroxy benzoic acids in the heartwood of the tree.[11] Several of these have strong microbicidal and fungicidal activities. Naphthoquinones are highly effective against *Candida albicans* and *Tricophyton mentagrophytes*.[12]

Lapachol has been shown to have antimicrobial[14] and antiviral[15] action. Beta-lapachone shows diversified antiparasitic activity[16] as well as antiviral action.[17] Alpha-lapachone is also active against some parasites,[18] and xyloidone is active against numerous bacteria and fungi.[19] Another LaPacho component, the flavonoid quercetin, is cytotoxic for some parasites.[20]

A wide array of organisms are effective against xyloidone. Several of the microorganisms are pathogenic, such as *Staphylococcus aureus* and the *Brucella* species. The causative agents of tuberculosis, dysentery, and anthrax are also inhibited by xyloidone. In addition to its activity against a variety of bacteria, this quinone inhibits several species of fungus, including *C. albicans*, *C. kruzei*, and *C. neoformans*.

Lapachol, like many naphthoquinones, interferes with energy production and enzymatic reactions with the microorganism.[22-32,57]

Antiviral activity

Lapachol, beta-lapachone, hydroxynapthoquinone, and other components of LaPacho have been shown to be active against a number of viruses, including herpes virus types I and II, influenza viruses, poliovirus, and vesicular stomatitis virus.[15,33]

Studies of beta-lapachone's antiviral activity have offered insights into the mechanism of this powerful quinone. Experiments with viruses demonstrated that beta-lapachone is able to inhibit some key viral enzymes, such as DNA and RNA polymerases, and retrovirus reverse transcriptase.[13] These actions have great significance in the possible treatment of AIDS, Epstein-Barr virus, and other viral infections.

Antiparasitic activity

The parasite *Schistosoma mansoni* is the causative agent of the common tropical disease schistosomiasis. The larva (cercariae) of this blood fluke live in water and enter the host by penetrating the skin. This debilitating disease, which is a serious problem in many tropical areas, weakens the host and increases susceptibility to a variety of other pathogens, some of which may be fatal.

Lapachol has been tested as a topical barrier to the cercariae and found to be highly effective at preventing its penetration.[34,35] Oral lapachol was also tested and found to significantly reduce penetration. After the lapachol was consumed, it was secreted into the skin, apparently by the sebaceous glands, where it again acted as a topical barrier. The cercariae seek to penetrate the host through or near the sebaceous glands, which suggests that dietary administration of lapachol would be an efficient means of protecting against infection.

Alpha-lapachone and beta-lapachone, also components of LaPacho, both exhibited activity against *S. mansoni*.[14] Another LaPacho component, beta-lapachone, is effective against *Trypanosoma cruzi*, the parasite responsible for trypanosomiasis, or Chaga's disease.[36,38] This disease occurs in both acute and chronic forms and is characterized in the acute form by swelling of the skin and enlargement of lymph nodes. In its chronic form it may affect the heart or nervous system.

Anticancer effects

Due to the folklore information surrounding the tumor-reducing qualities of LaPacho, this herb was extensively studied by the National Cancer Institute (NCI). Initially, results were positive.[45] Researchers believed that lapachol was the most active anticancer agent. Lapachol entered phase I clinical trials at NCI in 1968, based on its activity against Walker 256 tumors (with a confidence rate of over 90%). During these trials it was difficult to obtain therapeutic blood levels of lapachol without some mild toxic side effects such as nausea, vomiting, and anti-vitamin K activity. This is quite hard to understand because latter studies found the toxicity to be very low, with an LD_{50} of 487 mg/kg body weight—about the same as caffeine.[4] The Investigative New Drug (IND) status for the drug was closed in 1970.[45] It has been shown, however, that some of the anthraquinones in LaPacho have vitamin K activity. Therefore, use of the whole herb would compensate for lapachol's effect on vitamin K.[46]

The approach described indicates a flaw in the underlying philosophy of the pharmaceutical sciences and the NCI program. Because the initial studies came from a whole plant, the detailed studies should have been undertaken on the whole plant: some of the other components have also been shown to have anticancer activities.[37,39-44,47-55] Was it too complex to consider the chemical reactions of more than 20 components found in the LaPacho? Or did the standard economic/political incentive for patenting an analog impede the investigation of a plant species?

Lapachol is rapidly absorbed through the gastrointestinal tract after oral administration to rats bearing Walker 256 tumors. It is taken up by all tissues except the brain and blood cells. A significant amount appears in the tumor after 6 hr, with most of the drug disappearing from the other body tissue. The half-life of IV lapachol in mice is 33 min (75 min in dogs). Lapachol is metabolized extensively and excreted mostly in the feces.[1] Most other analogs had little effect on cancer.[48]

Anti-inflammatory activity

Extracts of the bark from *T. avellanedae* demonstrate clear anti-inflammatory activity with low toxicity.[21] Tampons soaked in an alcoholic extract of LaPacho have been shown to be very successful against a wide range of inflammations, such as cervicitis and cervicovaginitis.[2,13]

Summary

The spectrum of clinical applications of *T. avellanedae* is quite broad. Current use has focused on LaPacho's anticancer and antimicrobial activity. Its use is extremely popular in the treatment of intestinal candidiasis and vaginal candidiasis (topically and internally). There are also many anecdotal reports of remission of different forms of cancer from use of this botanical.[56]

Unfortunately, there has been a lack of quality control and confusion about the portion of the plant to use. (Many of the studies and chemical analyses have been done on the heartwood; yet, it is the bark that is available in the marketplace and discussed in the folklore.) Therefore, it is highly likely that most consumers and practitioners are not using effective materials, which could explain varying clinical results.

Dosage

The usual form of administration of LaPacho is as a decoction with the standard dose being 1 cup of decocted bark two to eight times a day. The decoction is made by boiling 1 tsp of LaPacho for each cup of water for 5–15 min.

A more precise dosage based on a lapachol content of 2–4% is 15–20 g of bark boiled in 500 ml or 1 pint water for 5–15 min three to four times a day.

Dosage of other forms (aqueous extract, fluid extract, solid extract) should be based on lapachol content, providing a daily lapachol intake of 1.5–2.0 g/day.

A tampon that has been soaked in the decoction or fluid extract is used in the treatment of vaginitis and cervicitis. The tampon is inserted vaginally and changed every 24 hr until resolution.

Toxicology

Although anti-vitamin K activity has been reported for lapachol, the presence of several vitamin K-like substances in the whole plant suggests this is not a problem. Lapachol has been reported to have an oral LD_{50} of 1.2–2.4 g/kg in albino rats and 487–621 mg/kg in mice.[5,8] In comparison, the oral LD_{50} of caffeine is 192 mg/kg in rats and 620 mg/kg in mice.[5]

Chronic administration of lapachol at a dose of 0.0625–0.25 g/kg/day to monkeys produces moderate to severe anemia. The anemia was most pronounced during the first 2 weeks of treatment. Death occurred in monkeys after six doses of lapachol at 0.5 g/kg/day and after five doses of 1.0 g/kg/day.[8]

There have been no reports in the literature of human toxicity when the whole bark is used as a decoction.

References

1. Willard T: Tabebuia Species. In: A Textbook of Natural Medicine. Pizzorno JE and Murray MT (eds.), JBC Publications, Seattle, WA, 1987 pp.Chapter V:Tabebuia

2. Burnett AR and Thomson RH: Naturally Occurring Quinones. Part X. The Quinonoid Constituents of Tabebuia avellanedae (Bignoniaceae), J Chem Soc (C) 1967. pp 2100-2104.

3. Pfizer C: Antitumor Composition from Lapachol and its Salts, CA70:9075B. 156

4. Canadian Health Protection Branch: Herbs and botanical preparations. Information Letter 726, Aug 13 1987

5. Duke JA: CRC Handbook of Medicinal Herbs. CRC Press, Inc, Boca Raton, Fl, 1985. pp470-3

6. Bernarde A: A Pocket Book of Brazilian Herbs (Folklore - History - Uses). Shogun Editora Rio de Janeiro Brazil, 1984. pp22-3

7. Hartwell JL: Plants used against cancer. A survey. Quarterman Publications, Lawrence, MA, 1982

8. Morrison RK, Brown DE, Oleson JJ, and Cooney DA: Oral toxicology studies with lapachol. Toxicol Appl Pharmacol 17:1-11, 1970

9. de Lima OG, d'Albuquerque IL, Machado MP, et al: Primeiras Observacoes sobre a acao antimicrobiana do lapachol. Anais da Sociedade de biologica de pernambuco XIV:129-35, 1956

10. de Lima OG, d'Albuquerque IL, Machado MP, et al: Uma Nova substancia Antibiotica isolada do "Pau D'Arco", Tabebuia sp. Anais da Sociedade de biologica de pernambuco XIV:136-40, 1956

11. Burnett AR and Thomson RH: Naturally occurring quinones. Part X. The Quinonoid Constituents of Tabebuia avellanedae (Bignoniaceae). J Chem Soc (C) 1967. pp2100-4

12. Gershon H and Shanks L: Fungitoxicity of 1,4-naphthoquinones to Candida albicans and Trichophyton mentagrophytes. Can J Microbiol 21:1317-21, 1975

13. Wanick MC, et al: Acao antiinflamatoria e cicatrizante do extrato hidroalcoolico do liber do pau d'arco roxo (Tabebuia avellanedae), em pacientes portadoras de cervicites e cervico-vaginites. Separata da Revista do Instituto de Antibioticos 10:41-6, 1970

14. de Lima OG, d'Albuquerque IL, Machado MP, et al: Primeiras Observacoes sobre a acao antimicrobiana do lapachol. Anais da Sociedade de biologica de pernambuco XIV:129-35, 1956

15. Lagrota M, et al: Antiviral activity of lapachol, Rev Microbiol 14:21-26, 1983

16. Lopes, J.N., Cruz, F.S., Docampo, R., Vasconcellos, M.E., Sampaio, C.R., Pinto, A.V., Gilbert, B. In vitro and in vivo evaluation of the toxicity of 1,4-naphthoquinone and 1,2-naphthoquinone derivatives against Trypanosoma cruzi. Ann Trop Med Parasit 72:523-01, 1978

17. Schuerch AR and Wehrli W: b-Lapachone, an inhibitor of oncornavirus reverse transcriptase and eukaryotic DNA polymerase-a: Inhibitory effect, thiol dependency and specificity. Eur J Biochem 84:197-205, 1978

18. Pinto AV, Pinto MDR and Gilbert B: Schistosomiasis mansoni: blockage of cercarial skin penetration by chemical agents: I. naphthoquinones and derivatives. Trans Royal Soc Trop Med Hyg 71:133-35, 1977

19. de Lima OG, d'Albuquerqul IL, de Lima CG, and Dalia Maia MII: Comunicacao XX. Antividade antimicrobiana de alguns derivados do lapachol em comparacao com a xiloidona, Nova ortonaftoquinona natural isolada de extractos do cerne do "Pau d'Arco" roxo, Tabebuia avellanedae Lor. ex. Griseb. Substancias antimicrobianas de plantas superiores. Revista do Instituto de Antibioticos Recife 4, 1962

20. Shapiro A, Nathan HC, Hutner SH, et al: In vivo and in vitro activity by diverse chelators against Trypanosoma brucei . J Protozool 29:85-90, 1982

21. Oga S and Sekino T: Toxicidade e Atividade Anti-inflamatoria de Tabebuia avellanedae Lorentz e Griesbach ("Ipe Roxo"). Rev Fac Farm Bioquim S Paulo 7:47-53, 1969

22. Howland JL: Uncoupling and inhibition of oxidative phosphorylation by 2-hydroxy-3-alkyl-1,4-naphthoquinones. Biochim Biophys Acta 77:659-62, 1963

23. Wendel WB: The influence of naphthoquinones upon the respiratory and carbohydrate metabolism of malarial parasites. Fed Proc 5:406-7, 1946

24. Ball EG, Anfinsen CB and Cooper O: The inhibitory action of naphthoquinones on respiratory processes. J Biol Chem 168:257-70, 1947

25. Fieser LF and Richardson AP: Naphthoquinone antimalarials. II. Correlation of structure and activity against Plasmodium lophurae in ducks. J Am Chem Soc 70:3156-65, 1948

26. Gosalvez M, Garcia-Canero R, Blanco M, and Guru charri-Lloyd C: Effects and specificity of anticancer agents on the respiration and energy metabolism of tumor cells. Canc Treat Rep 60:1-8, 1976

27. Crawford DR and Schneider DL: Identification of ubiquinone-50 in human neutrophils and its role in microbicidal events. J Biol Chem 257:6662-8, 1982

28. Wendel WB: The influence of naphthoquinones upon the respiratory and carbohydrate metabolism of malarial parasites. Fed Proc 5:406-7, 1946

29. Howland JL: Influence of alkylhydroxynaphthoquinones on the mitochondrial oxidation of tetramethyl-p-phenylenediamine. Biochim Biophys Acta 131:247-54, 1967

30. Hadler HI and Moreau TL: The induction of ATP energized mitochondrial volume changes by the combination of the two antitumour agents showdomycin and lapachol, J An tibiot 513-520, 1969

31. Douglas KT, et al: Lapachol inhibition of alpha-ketoaldehyde metabolism. IRCS Med Sci: Libr Compend 10:683, 1982
32. Koide SS: Inhibition of 3a-hydroxysteroid-mediated transhydrogenase of rat liver by various quinones and flavonoids. Biochim Biophys Acta 59:708-10, 1962
33. Linhares MIS and De Santana CF: Estudo sobre of efeito de substancias antibioticas obtidas de Streptomyces e veetais superiores sobre o Herpesvirus hominis. Revista Instituto Antibioticos, Recife 15:25-32, 1975
34. Austin FG: Schistosoma mansoni chemoprophylaxis with dietary lapachol. Am J Trop Med Hygiene 23:412-419, 1974
35. Gilbert B, de Souza JP, Fascio M, et al: Schistosomiasis. Protection against infection by terpenoids. An Acad Brasil Cienc 42(supl):397-400, 1970
36. Goijman SG and Stoppani AOM: Oxygen radicals and macromolecule turnover in Trypanosoma cruzi. Life Chem Rep suppl 2, 1984. pp216-21
37. Docampo R, Cruz FS, Boveris A, et al: b-Lapachone enhancement of lipid peroxidation and superoxide anion and hydrogen peroxide formation by sarcoma 180 ascites tumor cells. Biochem Pharmacol 28:723-8, 1979
38. Boveris A, Stoppani AOM, Docampo R, and Cruz FS: Superoxide anion production and trypanocidal action of naphthoquinones on Trypanosoma cruzi. Comp Biochem Phys 327-9, 1978
39. Schaffner-Sabba K, et al: b-Lapachone: Synthesis of derivatives and activities in tumour models. J Medicinal Chem 27:990-4, 1984
40. Graziani Y, The effect of quercetin of pp60v-src kinase activities. Plant Flavonoids in Biology and Medicine: Biochemical, Pharmacological, and Structure-Activity Relationships. Alan R Liss, Inc, 1986. pp301-13
41. Hodnick WF, et al: Inhibition of mitochondrial respiration and production of superoxide and hydrogen peroxide by flavonoids: A structure activity study. Plant Flavonoids in Biology and Medicine: Biochemical, Pharmacological, and Structure-Activity Relationships. Alan R Liss, Inc, 1986. pp249-52
42. Srivastava AK, et al: Effect of quercetin on serine/threonine and tyrosine protein kinases. Plant Flavonoids in Biology and Medicine: Biochemical, Pharmacological, and Structure-Activity Relationships. Alan R Liss, Inc, 1986. pp315-8
43. Pizzorno JE and Murray MT: A Textbook of Natural Medicine. Pizzorno JE and Murray MT (eds.), JBC Publications, Seattle, WA, 1987 pp.Chapter V:Quercetin
44. Selway JWT: Antiviral activity of flavones and flavins. Plant Flavonoids in Biology and Medicine: Biochemical, Pharmacological, and Structure-Activity Relationships. Alan R Liss, Inc, 1986. pp521-36
45. Block JB, Serpick AA, Miller W, and Wiernik PH: Early clinical studies with lapachol (NSC-11905). Cancer Chemo Rep 4:27-8, 1974
46. Preusch PC and Suttie J W: Lapachol inhibition of vitamin K epoxide reductase and vitamin K quinone reductase. Arch Biochem Biophys 234:405-12, 1984
47. McKelvey EM, Lomedica M, Lu K, et al: Dichloroallyl lawsone. Clin Pharmacol Ther 586-590, 1979
48. Rao KV: Quinone natural products: Streptonigrin (NSC-45383) and lapachol (NSC-11905) structure-activity relationships. Cancer Chemo Rep 4:11-7, 1974
49. Ball EG: Studies on oxidation-reduction. XXII: Lapachol, lomatiol, and related compounds. J Biol Chem 114:649-55, 1936
50. Ball EG, Anfinsen CB and Cooper O: The inhibitory action of naphthoquinones on respiratory processes. J Biol Chem 168:257-70, 1947
51. Bachur NR, Gordon SL, Gee MV: NADPH cytochrome P-450 reductase activation of quinone anticancer agents to free radicals. Proc Natl Acad Sci USA 76:954-57, 1979
52. Bachur NR, Gordon SL, and Gee MV: A general mechanism for microsomal activation of quinone anticancer agents to free radicals. Cancer Res 38:1745-50, 1978
53. Iwamoto Y, Hansen IL, Porter TH, and Folkers K: Inhibition of coenzyme Q10-enzymes, succinoxidase and NADH-oxidase, by adriamycin and other quinones having antitumor activity. Biochem Biophys Res Comm 58:633-8, 1974
54. Bennett LL, Smithers D, Rose LM, et al: Inhibition of synthesis of pyrimidine nucleotides by 2-hydroxy-3-(3,3-dichloroallyl)-1,4-naphthoquinone. Cancer Res 39:4868-74, 1979
55. Lee S-H, Sutherland TO, Deves R, and Brodie AF: Respiration of /active transport of solutes and oxidative phosphorylation by naphthoquinones in irradiatiated membrane vesicle from Mycobacterium phlei. Proc Natl Acad Sci USA 77:102-6, 1980
56. Weed B: Second Opinion, Lapacho fight against cancer. Rostrum Communication, Vancouver, Canada, 1984
57. Ball EG: Studies on oxidation-reduction. XXII. Lapachol, Lomatiol, and related compounds. J Biol Chem 114:649-55, 1936

SECTION V

Herbs for the heart and vascular system

$\mathbf{A}$therosclerotic cardiovascular disease remains the number one killer of Americans. Elevated blood pressure is one of the major contributors to this disease. Hypertension, or high blood pressure, affects over 20% of the adult white population and over 30% of the adult black population. Because hypertension is a major risk factor for cardiovascular related death, physicians have sought ways of effectively lowering blood pressure. Despite the fact that diet alone has been shown to be equally as effective as many drug therapies, the majority of patients are given prescription drugs. These drugs, however, may be placing the patients in an early grave because several long-term studies have indicated that taking medications designed to lower blood pressure may actually increase the risk of having a heart attack. Most notably among these medications are the diuretics and beta-blockers.

Beta-blockers, like propranolol (trade name Inderal), are one of the most widely prescribed drugs in the United States. They act in lowering blood pressure by decreasing heart rate and cardiac output. These drugs have many known side effects, including congestive heart failure, lightheadedness, depression, fatigue, and sexual impotence. Beta-blockers are known to increase levels of cholesterol and triglycerides in the blood. This effect probably explains why patients on beta-blockers have a higher incidence of heart attacks than high-risk patients not on any medications.

Diuretics have also been shown to increase the risk of having a heart attack. Diuretics promote the excretion of minerals like calcium and magnesium. These two minerals have been shown to be effective agents in lowering elevated blood pressures and in preventing heart attacks.

The irony is that nondrug treatment is supported by most authorities, especially for mild to moderate hypertension (diastolic <95 mmHg). Numerous studies have concluded that harmful side effects of beta-blockers and diuretics outweighed the therapeutic benefits of these agents and supported effective life-style changes as safe alternatives. Most authorities, including the Joint National Committee on Detection, Evaluation and Treatment of High Blood Pressure, are now recommending that the majority of hypertensive patients not be placed on drugs.

The best treatment of high blood pressure appears to be making life-style and dietary changes that will lower blood pressure. The most important nutritional factor appears to be achieving normal body weight, which often results in normalization of blood pressure. A high-fiber, low-fat, low-sodium diet has been shown to be as effective in reducing blood pressure as beta-blockers and/or diuretics.

The life-style factors that appear to contribute most significantly to hypertension are smoking, stress levels, and alcohol consumption. If additional support is needed, nutritional supplements and botanical medicines such as *Crataegus oxyacantha* or *Coleus forskohlii* may be used. These two botanicals, along with gugulipid and *Ginkgo biloba*, are discussed in this important section.

Gugulipid is a remarkable cholesterol-lowering herbal compound from India; *G. biloba* may be the most important medicinal plant on this planet. Ginkgo is being hailed as a "miracle drug" in Europe and is currently the most widely prescribed medicine in France and Germany.

14

Hawthorn

(CRATAEGUS OXYACANTHA)

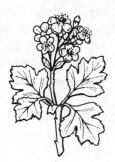

Key uses of hawthorn:

- Atherosclerosis
- High blood pressure
- Congestive heart failure
- Angina

General description

Crataegus oxyacantha is a spiny tree or shrub that is native to Europe. It may reach a height of 30 ft but is often grown as a hedge. Its common name, hawthorn, is actually a corruption of "hedgethorn"; it was used in Germany to divide plots of land. Its botanical name is from the Greek *kratos*, meaning "hardness" (of the wood), *oxus* meaning "sharp," and *akantha* meaning "a thorn." The fruit and blossoms are used medicinally.[1]

Other species of hawthorn—e.g., *C. monogyna* and *C. pentagyna*—have similar pharmacological actions to *C. oxyacantha* and are suitable alternatives.[2,3]

Chemical composition

Hawthorn leaves, berries, and blossoms contain many biologically active flavonoid compounds, particularly anthocyanidins and proanthocyanidins (polymers of anthocyanidins, also known as biflavans or procyanidins).[4,5] These flavonoids are responsible for the red to blue colors not only of hawthorn berries but also of blackberries, cherries, blueberries, grapes, and many flowers. These compounds are highly concentrated in hawthorn berry and flower extracts.

High-performance liquid chromatography and thin-layer chromatography have demonstrated that extracts of the flowers are particularly rich in flavonoids (quercetin, quercetin-3-galactoside, vitexin, vitexin-4'-rhamnoside, etc.) and proanthocyanidins.[5,6]

Hawthorn extracts also contain cardiotonic amines (e.g., phenylethylamine, o-methoxyphenylethylamine, tyramine, isobutylamine); choline and acetylcholine; purine derivatives (e.g., adenosine, adenine, guanine, and caffeic acid); amygdalin; pectins; and triterpene acids (ursolic, oleonolic, and crategolic acids).[7]

History and folk use

Hawthorn flowers and berries have been used primarily as cardiac tonics and mild diuretics in organic and functional heart disorders. They have also been used for their astringent qualities, to relieve the discomfort of sore throats.[1]

Pharmacology

The pharmacology of hawthorn centers on its flavonoid components. The proanthocyanidins in hawthorn are largely responsible for its cardiovascular activities.

Synergism with vitamin C

Crataegus is particularly rich in anthocyanidins and proanthocyanidins. These flavonoids have very strong "vitamin P" activity. They are able to increase intracellular vitamin C levels, stabilize vitamin C (by protecting it from destruction or oxidation), and decrease capillary permeability and fragility.[4,8,9]

Collagen-stabilizing action

The flavonoid components of hawthorn have significant collagen-stabilizing action. Collagen is the most abundant protein of the body and is responsible for maintaining the integrity of ground substance, tendons, ligaments, and cartilage. Collagen is destroyed during inflammatory processes that occur in rheumatoid arthritis, periodontal disease, and other inflammatory conditions that involve bones, joints, cartilage, and other connective tissue. Anthocyanidins, proanthocyanidins, and other flavonoids are remarkable in their ability to prevent collagen destruction. They affect collagen metabolism in many ways, including:

1. The unique ability to actually crosslink collagen fibers, resulting in reinforcement of the natural crosslinking of collagen that forms the collagen matrix of connective tissue (ground substance, cartilage, tendon, etc.)[4,8,9]
2. The prevention of free radical damage, due to potent and free radical scavenging action[4,8-10]
3. The inhibition of enzymatic cleavage by enzymes secreted by white blood cells during inflammation[4,8,9]
4. The prevention of the release and synthesis of compounds that promote inflammation, such as prostaglandins, serine proteases, histamine, and leukotrienes[9-12]

These effects on collagen and their potent antioxidant activity make hawthorn extracts extremely useful in the treatment of a wide variety of inflammatory conditions. Hawthorn berries, like cherries,[13] are particularly effective in the treatment of gout because their flavonoid components are able to reduce uric acid levels as well as reduce tissue destruction.

Cardiovascular effects

Hawthorn extracts are effective in reducing blood pressure, angina attacks, and serum cholesterol levels and in preventing the deposition of cholesterol in arterial walls.[2,14,15] Hawthorn extracts are widely used in Europe and Asia for their antihypertensive and cardiotonic activity. The beneficial pharmacological effects of hawthorn in the treatment of these conditions appears to be a result of the following actions:

1. Improvement of the blood supply to the heart by dilating the coronary vessels[2,14,16-19]
2. Improvement of the metabolic processes in the heart, which results in an increase in the force of contraction of the heart muscle and elimination of some types of rhythm disturbances[2,14,20-22]
3. Inhibition of angiotensin converting enzyme (ACE)[23]

Hawthorn's ability to dilate coronary blood vessels, the vessels supplying the heart with vital oxygen and nutrients, has been repeatedly demonstrated in experimental studies.[2,14,16-19] This effect appears to be due to relaxation of the smooth muscle components of the vessel. Various flavonoid components in *Crataegus* have been shown to inhibit constriction of vessels by a variety of substances.[2,8,9] When blood vessels constrict, blood pressure goes up. In addition, procyanidins have been shown to inhibit angiotensin converting enzyme (ACE).[23] This enzyme is responsible for converting angiotensin I to angiotensin II, which is a potent constrictor of blood vessels.

Recently, several proanthocyanidins have demonstrated a specific inhibition of ACE similar to that of captopril.[23] Captopril is a synthetic ACE inhibitor widely used in the treatment of high blood pressure. The proanthocyanidins that appear to have the highest activity are those found in relatively high concentrations in hawthorn berries, flowers, and their extracts.[4,5]

Improvement in energy production within the heart has been demonstrated in humans and animals to whom hawthorn extracts have been administered.[2,14,20,21] The improvement is a result not only of increased blood and oxygen supply to the myocardium (muscle of the heart) but also of flavonoid-enzyme interactions. In particular, hawthorn extracts and various flavonoid components in *Crataegus* have been shown to inhibit several key enzymes within the myocardium (e.g., cyclic adenosine monophosphate phosphodiesterase).[22] This net result is an increase in the force of contraction, which is particularly beneficial in cases of congestive heart failure.

Atherosclerosis

Hawthorn berries or extracts should be thought of as a necessary food in the prevention and treatment of atherosclerosis. Increasing the intake of flavonoid compounds through hawthorn extracts has numerous health-promoting effects, including reducing cholesterol levels and decreasing the size of existing atherosclerotic plaques.[15] This again is probably a result of collagen stabilization.

A decrease in the integrity of the collagen matrix of the artery results in cholesterol deposits within the artery. Many researchers feel that if the collagen matrix of the artery remains strong, the atherosclerotic plaque will never develop. *Crataegus* flavonoids, by increasing the integrity of collagen structures, may offer significant protection against atherosclerosis. It may even reverse the effects of early atherosclerotic activity. In some experiments, feeding proanthocyanidin extracts to animals has resulted in reversal of atherosclerotic lesions, as well as decreased serum cholesterol levels.[15]

Flavonoids contained in hawthorn extracts appear to offer significant prevention, as well as potential reversing effects, in the treatment of atherosclerotic processes, which are still the major causes of death in the United States.

Hypertension

Crataegus exerts a mild antihypertensive effect, demonstrated in many experimental and clinical studies. Its action in lowering blood pressure is unique in that it does so through a number of diverse pharmacological effects. Specifically, it dilates the coronary vessels, inhibits ACE, increases the functional capacity of the heart, and has a mild diuretic action.

The effects of hawthorn generally require prolonged administration, and in many instances it may take up to 2 weeks before adequate tissue concentrations are achieved.

Beta-blockers (e.g., Inderal) lower blood pressure by reducing cardiac output. Keep in mind that administering hawthorn to patients taking beta-blockers may produce a mild hypertensive response by increasing cardiac output.

Congestive heart failure

Crataegus has a long history of use in the treatment of congestive heart failure (CHF), particularly in combination with digitalis or other herbs that contain cardiac glycosides (e.g., *Cereus grandifloris*, also known as *Cactus grandifloris*, and *Convallaria majalis*). It potentiates the action of the cardiac glycosides.

Because of this enhancing effect, lower doses of cardiac glycosides can be used. In addition, magnesium has also been shown to augment digitalis action. For mild to moderate cases of CHF, *Crataegus* extract used alone may be sufficient, but for moderate to severe CHF, it should be used in combination with other cardiac glycosides as prescribed by a health care professional.

Summary

Crataegus berries and extracts are useful as food supplements in conditions that affect collagen structures, such as arthritis, periodontal disease, atherosclerosis, and inflammation. *Crataegus* extracts also demonstrate very beneficial effects on the heart and blood vessels. This plant has been used successfully in the treatment of hypertension, cardiac arrythmias, congestive heart failure, and angina. Its pharmacological activity is related to its high content of flavonoid compounds.

Dosage

The dosage depends on the type of preparation and source material. Standardized extracts, similar to those used in Europe and Asia as prescription medications, are available commercially. The doses listed for the various formulas are for use three times a day:

- Hawthorn berries or flowers (dried)—3–5 g or as an infusion
- Hawthorn tincture (1:5)—4–6 ml (1–1½ tsp (Note: Alcohol may elicit pressor response in some individuals.)

- Hawthorn fluid extract (1:1)—1–2 ml ($\frac{1}{4}$–$\frac{1}{2}$ tsp)
- Hawthorn freeze dried berries—1–1.5 g
- Hawthorn flower extract (standardized to contain 1.8% vitexin-4'-rhamnoside or 10% procyanidins)—100–250 mg

Toxicology

Crataegus has been shown to have low toxicity. In rats, the typical acute LD_{50} of the tincture is about 25 ml/kg for oral administration; toxicity for chronic administration is found at about 5 ml/kg.[14] Similar results, adjusted for concentration, are found with other forms of *Crataegus*.

Although some studies have shown that proanthocyanidins may be carcinogenic, more careful evaluation has indicated that the carcinogenicity was probably due to nitrosamines found in the extracts used.[24] Purified proanthocyanidins have been found to be nonmutagenic, according to the *Salmonella* mutagenicity assay system (Ames test).[24]

References

1. Grieve M: A Modern Herbal, Vol 1. Dover Publications, New York, NY, 1971. pp385-6
2. Petkov V: Plants with hypotensive, antiatheromatous and coronarodilating action. Am J Chin Med 7:197-236, 1979
3. Thompson EB, Aynilian GH, Gora P, and Farnsworth NR: Preliminary study of potential antiarrhythmic effects of Crataegus monogyna. J Pharm Sci 63:1936-7, 1974
4. Kuhnau J: The flavonoids: A class of semi-essential food components: Their role in human nutrition. Wld Rev Nutr Diet 24:117-91, 1976
5. Ficarra P, Ficarra R, Tommasini A, et al: High-performance liquid chromatography of flavonoids in Crataegus oxyacantha. Il Farmaco Ed Pr 39:148-57, 1983
6. Wagner H, Bladt S and Zgainski EM: Plant Drug Analysis. Springer-Verlag, New York, NY 1984. pp166,178,179
7. Wagner H and Grevel J: Cardiotonic drugs IV, cardiotonic amines from Crataegus oxyacantha. Planta Medica 45:98-101, 1982
8. Gabor M: Pharmacologic effects of flavonoids on blood vessels. Angiologica 9:355-74, 1972
9. Havsteen B: Flavonoids, a class of natural products of high pharmacological potency. Biochem Pharm 32:1141-8, 1983
10. Middleton E: The flavonoids. Trends Pharm Sci 5:335-8, 1984
11. Amella M, Bronner C, Briancon F, et al: Inhibition of mast cell histamine release by flavonoids and bioflavonoids. Planta Medica 51:16-20, 1985
12. Busse WW, Kopp DE and Middleton E: Flavonoid modulation of human neutrophil function. J Allergy Clin Immunol 73:801-9, 1984
13. Blau LW: Cherry diet control for gout and arthritis. Tex Rep Biol Med 8:309-11, 1950
14. Ammon HPT and Handel M: Crataegus, toxicology and pharmacology. Planta Medica 43:101-120,318-22, 1981
15. Wegrowski J, Robert AM and Moczar M: The effect of procyanidolic oligomers on the composition of normal and hypercholesterolemic rabbit aortas. Biochem Pharm 33:3491-7, 1984
16. Mavers VWH and Hensel H: Changes in local myocardial blood flow following oral administration to a crataegus extract to non-anesthetized dogs. Arzniem Forsch 24:783-5, 1974
17. Roddewig VC and Hensel H: Reaction of local myocardial blood flow in non-anesthetized dogs and

anesthetized cats to oral and parenteral application of a crataegus fraction (oligomere procyanidins). Arzneim Forsch 27:1407-10, 1977

18. Rewerski VW, Piechocki T, Tyalski M, and Lewak S: Some pharmacological properties of oligomeric procyanidin isolated from hawthorn (Crataegus oxyacantha). Arzniem Forsch 17:490-1, 1967
19. Hammerl H, Kranzl C, Pichler O, and Studlar M: Klinixch-experimentelle toffwechselunter-suchungen mit einem crataegus-extrakt. Arzniem Forsch 21:261-3, 1971
20. Vogel VG: Predictability of the activity of drug combinations - yes or no? Arzniem Forsch 25:1356-65, 1975
21. O'Conolly VM, Jansen W, Bernhoft G, and Bartsch G: Treatment of cardiac performance (NYHA stages I to II) in advanced age with standardized crataegus extract. Fortschr Med 104:805-8, 1986
22. Petkov E, Nikolov N and Uzunov P: Inhibitory effect of some flavonoids and flavonoid mixtures on cyclic AMP phosphodiesterase activity of rat heart. Planta Medica 43:183-6, 1981
23. Uchida S, Ikari N, Ohta H, et al: Inhibitory effects of condensed tannins on angiotensin converting enzyme. Jap J Pharmacol 43:242-5, 1987
24. Yu Cl and Swaminathan B: Mutagenicity of proanthocyanidins. Food Chem Toxicol 25:135-9, 1987

15

Coleus

(COLEUS FORSKOHLII)

Key uses of coleus:

- High blood pressure
- Angina
- Psoriasis
- Asthma and allergies

General description

Coleus forskohlii is a small member of the Lamiaceae (mint) family, which grows as a perennial in India. It is cultivated as an ornamental plant, and the root is used for medicinal purposes and as a condiment.

Chemical composition

The root contains an essential oil and diterpenes that exhibit pharmacological activity. Forskolin concentration is typically 0.2–0.3%. No other species of coleus contains forskolin.

History and folk use

Coleus has been used since antiquity in Hindu and Ayurvedic traditional medicine and is the source of an amazing compound of unique biological importance—a compound known as forskolin. While the majority of studies about the medicinal effects of coleus have been done using forskolin, it is believed that other components within the plant extract may enhance the absorption and biological activity of forskolin. The pharmacological activity of this compound is, however, substantiating the traditional uses of the herb, which includes such things as heart disease, abdominal colic, respiratory disorders, painful urination, insomnia, and convulsions.[1]

In 1974 pharmacological screening of medicinal plants by the Indian Central Drug Research Institute revealed that extracts of coleus roots have significant blood pressure lowering and antispasmodic effects. The active constituent was isolated and named coleonol (later renamed forskolin).

Pharmacology

The basic mechanism of forskolin is the activation of the enzyme adenylate cyclase, which increases the cyclic adenosine monophosphate (AMP) in cells.[2] Cyclic AMP is perhaps the most important cell-regulating compound. Once formed, it activates many other enzymes involved in diverse cellular functions.

The physiological and biochemical effects of increased intracellular cyclic AMP are numerous. They include relaxation of smooth muscle; inhibition of platelet activation, mast cell degranulation, and basophil release; increased force of heart-muscle contraction; and increased lipolysis in adipocytes.

There are many conditions in which a decreased intracellular cyclic AMP level is thought to be a major factor in the development of the disease. *C. forskohlii* appears to be extremely well indicated for eczema (atopic dermatitis), asthma, psoriasis, angina, and hypertension.

Smooth muscle relaxing effects

Forskolin has been shown to have tremendous antispasmodic action on smooth muscles.[1,3,4] This supports the long-time use of *C. forskohlii* in the treatment of intestinal colic, asthma, uterine cramps (menstrual cramps), painful urination, angina, and hypertension.

Cardiovascular effects

The cardiovascular effects of *C. forskohlii* and its components have been studied in great detail.[1,3,7] Its basic cardiovascular actions involve lowering of blood pressure, along with improved contractility of the heart. Again, this is related to increasing cyclic AMP levels throughout the cardiovascular system, which results in relaxation of the arteries and increased force of contraction. The net effect is tremendous improvement in cardiovascular function.

C. forskohlii extract, alone or in combination with other botanicals (e.g., *Crataegus* and *Ammi visnaga*) is indicated for virtually all cardiovascular complaints, particularly hypertension, congestive heart failure, and angina.

Action in allergic conditions

Atopic allergic conditions such as asthma and eczema are characterized by a relative decrease in cyclic AMP in the bronchial smooth muscle and skin, respectively. Current drug therapy for these conditions is designed to increase cyclic AMP levels by inhibiting enzymes that break down cyclic AMP once it is formed. This is different than forskolin's ability to increase the initial production of cyclic AMP through activating the enzyme adenylate cyclose.

Increasing cellular levels of cyclic AMP results in relaxation of bronchial muscles and relief of asthma symptoms. Forskolin has been shown to have remarkable effects in relaxing constricted bronchial muscles in asthmatics,[4,5] most likely due to an increase in cyclic AMP, although forskolin has other antiallergic activities, such as inhibiting the release of histamine and the synthesis of allergic compounds.[6]

Action in psoriasis

Psoriasis is an extremely common skin disorder that seems to be caused by a relative decrease in cyclic AMP when compared to another cell-regulating compound, cyclic guanine monophosphate (GMP). The result is a tremendous increase in cell division. In fact, cells divide in psoriasis at a rate 1,000 times greater than normal. Preliminary studies indicate that forskolin may be of great benefit to individuals with psoriasis because it normalizes the balance that exists between cyclic AMP and cyclic GMP.[1]

The future of forskolin

Forskolin, because of its unique ability to increase cyclic AMP levels by activating adenylate cyclase, has become an invaluable aid in learning how cellular processes are regulated.[2] Forskolin has provided many answers to puzzling questions over the past 10 years and will continue to do so in the future. In addition, forskolin will probably be synthesized and marketed as a drug in the near future. For most uses, the crude plant extract may offer better results. However, there are a couple of indications that may be better served by the isolated constituent. Specifically, forskolin may prove to be of tremendous value in the acute treatment of glaucoma and asthma.

In clinical studies, forskolin was shown to greatly reduce intraocular pressure when it was applied directly to the eyes. This result indicates that the compound may be of great benefit in the treatment of glaucoma.[8,9] Forskolin, administered as an aerosol, has been shown to prevent asthma attacks. It is available in this form in Europe.[10] During an acute attack, an asthmatic needs immediate relief. It appears that the aerosol-administered forskolin may offer this immediate relief.

Summary

The ancient medicinal plant *C. forskohlii* is the source of the compound forskolin, which possesses unique biological activity. Research upholds the traditional uses of the plant extract by investigating the pharmacological effects of forskolin. Although clinical results are thought to be better obtained using the whole plant, the isolated constituent (forskolin) may become a widely utilized drug in the treatment of a wide variety of conditions. At present, *C. forskohlii* extracts appear to be indicated in cases of hypertension, congestive heart failure, angina, asthma, eczema, and psoriasis.

Dosage

The following dosages are for three times a day:

- Dried plant—3–5 g or as an infusion
- *C. forskohlii* tincture (1:5)—4–6 ml (1–1½ tsp)
- *C. forskohlii* fluid extract (1:1)—1–2 ml (¼–½ tsp)
- *C. forskohlii* extract (4:1)—200–400 mg

Toxicology

No adverse reactions to *C. forskohlii* could be found in the scientific literature.

References

1. Ammon HPT and Muller AB: Forskolin: from Ayurvedic remedy to a modern agent. Planta Medica 51:473-7, 1985
2. Seamon KB and Daly JW: Forskolin: a unique diterpene activator of cyclic AMP-generating systems. J Cyclic Nucleotide Research 7:201-24, 1981
3. Dubey MP, Srimal RC, Nityand S and Dhawan BN: Pharmacological studies on coleonol, a hypotensive diterpene from Coleus forskohlii. J Ethnopharmacology 3:1-13, 1981
4. Kreutner W, Chapman RW, Gulbenkian A and Tozzi S: Bronchodilato and antiallergy activity of forskolin. European J Pharmacology 111:1-8, 1985
5. Kerouac R, St-Pierre S and Rioux F: Forskolin inhibits histamine release by neurotensin in the rat perfused hind limb. Research Communications Chemical Pathology Pharmacology 45:310-2, 1984
6. Chang J, Cherney ML, Moyer JA and Lewis AJ: Effect of forskolin on prostaglandin on prostaglandin synthesis by mouse resident peritoneal macrophages. European J Pharmacology 103:303-12, 1984
7. Lindner E, Dohadwalla AN and Bhattacharya BK: Positive inotropic and blood pressure lowering activity of a diterpene derivative isolated from Coleus forskohli: forskolin. Arzneim.-Forsch 28:284-9, 1978
8. Potter DE, Burke JA and Temple JR: Forskolin suppresses sympathetic neuron function and causes ocular hypotension. Current Eye Research 4:87-96, 1985
9. Caprioli J and Sears M: Forskolin lowers intraocular pressure in rabbits, monkeys, and man. Lancet i:958-60, 1983
10. Lichey J, Friedrich T, Priesnitz M, et al: Effect of forskolin on methacholine-induced bronchoconstriction in extrinsic asthmatics. Lancet ii:167, 1984

16

Ginkgo biloba

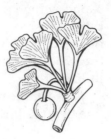

Key uses of *Ginkgo biloba:*

- Decreased blood supply to the brain
- Senility, ringing in the ears, dizziness
- Impotence
- Varicose veins
- Alzheimer's disease

General description

Ginkgo biloba is a deciduous tree that may live as long as 1,000 years, growing to a height of 100–122 ft and a diameter of 3–4 ft. The ginkgo has short horizontal branches with short shoots, bearing leaves that measure 5–10 cm across. The leaf resembles a fan or the maidenhair fern, which is why the ginkgo has been called the "maidenhair tree." It is the leaves of the ginkgo that are used medicinally.

Ginkgo bears a foul-smelling, nonedible fruit and an ivory-colored inner seed that resembles an almond. The seed is edible and is sold in marketplaces in the Orient.

Chemical composition

The active components of ginkgo leaves are the so-called ginkgo heterosides, or ginkgo-flavone glycosides (flavonoid molecules that are unique to the ginkgo), several terpene molecules unique to ginkgo (ginkgolides and bilobalide), and organic acids.[1]

The *G. biloba* extract (GBE) marketed in Europe under the trade names Tanakan, Rokan, and Tebonin is a very well defined and complex product prepared from the green leaves. The mode of culture, harvesting, and extraction are perfectly standardized and controlled.

GBE is standardized to contain 24% flavonoid glycosides. These molecules represent a convenient analytical reference group for primary standardization of the extract. Although they do play a major role in the pharmacological activity of GBE, other components are also important.

The ginkgo flavonoid glycoside contains an aglycone (flavonoid) portion bound to a glucoside (sugar) component. The three major aglycones are quercetin, kaempferol, and isorhamnetin. The glucosidic components are glucose and rhamnose, present as monoglucosides or diglucosides, in esterified as well as nonesterified forms.

Other significant flavonoid components of the extract include proanthocyanidins, largely composed of dimers and oligomers of delphinidine and cyanidin.

The major terpene molecules of GBE are the diterpene ginkgolides and the sesquiterpene bilobalide. These compounds are unique to ginkgo and are not found in any other plants. They account for 6% of the extract.

The three major ginkgolides present are termed ginkgolide A, B, and C. These compounds differ by the presence of one, two, or three hydroxyl groups respectively. Bilobalide is a trilactone that possesses a tertiary butyl group.

Other constituents of GBE include a number of organic acids (hydroxykinurenic, kynurenic, protocatechic, vanillic, etc.). These compounds contribute valuable properties to the extract by making the usually water-insoluble flavonoid and terpene molecules of ginkgo water-soluble.

History and folk use

G. biloba is the world's oldest living tree species. It is the sole survivor of the family Ginkgoaceae. Because the ginkgo tree can be traced back more than 200 million years to the fossils of the Permian period, it is often referred to as the "living fossil." Once common in North America and Europe, the ginkgo was almost destroyed during the Ice Age. It was destroyed in all regions of the world except China. It has long been cultivated in China as a sacred tree.

In the late 17th century, Dr. Engelbert Kaempfer, a German physician and botanist, became the first European to discover and catalog the ginkgo tree. The flavonoid kaempferol is named for Kaempfer. In 1771, Linnaeus named the tree *Ginkgo biloba*.

The ginkgo tree was brought to the United States in 1784, to the garden of William Hamilton near Philadelphia. This tree species is now planted throughout much of the United States as an ornamental tree. The ginkgo is highly resistant to insects, disease, and pollution and thus is frequently planted along city streets.[1]

G. *biloba*'s medicinal use can be traced back to the oldest Chinese *materia medica* (2800 B.C.). The leaves have been used in traditional Chinese medicine for their ability to "benefit the brain," relieve the symptoms of asthma and coughs, and help the body eliminate filaria, the worm that causes elephantitis.

Ginkgo leaf extracts are now the leading prescription medicines in both Germany and France, accounting for 1.0% and 1.5% of total prescription sales in Germany and France, respectively.[2] More than 100,000 physicians worldwide wrote more than 10 million prescriptions in 1989.

Pharmacology

The standardized concentrated extract of the leaves of G. *biloba* (24% ginkgo heteroside content) has demonstrated remarkable pharmacologic effects. According to Drieu, the total extract is more active than single isolated components, which suggests synergism between the various components of GBE.[1] This notion is well supported in more than 250 clinical and experimental studies that used the extract. However, recently there has been much interest in the ginkgolides and bilobalide.

Pharmacokinetics

The pharmacokinetics of GBE has been studied in rats using radiolabeled carbon (^{14}C).[15] It must be pointed out that the analytical study of the tagged extract showed that the ^{14}C radioactivity was not uniformly distributed among the various constituents of the extract. Radioactivity was limited largely to the flavonoid components. No radioactivity was found in the terpenes nor in the principle sugars after hydrolysis of the glycosides.

Following oral administration, absorption of the radiolabeled extract was at least 60%. Because blood levels peaked after 1.5 hr, researchers suspect upper gastrointestinal tract absorption.

During the first 3 hr, radioactivity was primarily associated with the plasma. Progressively, erythrocytes will uptake the radiolabeled material so that at 48 hr it has equilibrated with the plasma.

The flavonoids appear to have an affinity for organs rich in connective tissues, such as the aorta, eyes, skin, and lungs. Levels of radioactivity in these tissues are two to three times higher than that in plasma and decreases little over the course of time. In the heart, specific activity retained is twice that retained in the skeletal muscles.

Radioactivity in the hippocampus and striated bodies of the brain at 72 hr show radioactivity five times greater than that of the plasma. The deposition pattern is similar to results from the circulation improvement observed after oxygen deprivation due to blood clots in rats. Other areas of the brain such as the cerebral cortex, brainstem, and cerebellum do not show such high levels of radioactivity. The adrenal glands retained the greatest level of radioactivity among the body's glands.

General tissue effects

GBE exerts profound general tissue effects, including membrane-stabilizing, antioxidant, and free radical scavenging effects.[3] GBE also enhances the utilization of oxygen and glucose.[4,5]

Cellular membranes are the first line of defense in the integrity of the cell. Largely composed of phospholipids, cellular membranes also serve as fluid barriers, exchange sites, and electrical capacitors.

Cell membranes are fragile and vulnerable. They are especially susceptible to lipid peroxidation induced by oxygenated free radicals. GBE is an extremely effective inhibitor of lipid peroxidation of cellular membranes.[6]

Erythrocytes (red blood cells) provide the best models for evaluating the effects of substances on membranal functions because the erythrocyte ion transport systems are well described; there is only a single intracellular ion compartment, and both intracellular and extracellular ionic concentrations can be easily determined. Studies have demonstrated that in addition to stabilizing membrane structures directly and enhancing free radical scavenging effects, GBE also activates membranal Na^+K^+ATP-ase, or sodium pump.[3,7] This enzyme is responsible for the exchange of intracellular sodium for extracellular potassium. In essence, GBE leads to better membranal polarization, which is extremely important in excitable tissues, particularly nerve tissues.

Neuronal cells

The membrane-stabilizing and free radical scavenging effects of GBE are perhaps most evident in the central nervous system. Brain cells contain the highest percentage of unsaturated fatty acids in their membranes of any cells in the body, making them extremely susceptible to lipid peroxidation.

The brain cell is also extremely susceptible to low oxygen levels. Unlike most tissues, the brain has very few energy reserves. The functions and homeostasis of the brain require a great amount of energy, which must be supplied by a constant availability of glucose and oxygen. When cerebral circulation diminishes, it sets up a chain of reactions that disrupt membrane function and energy production. The chain of reactions ultimately leads to cellular death.

GBE has a remarkable ability to prevent metabolic and neuronal disturbances in experimental models of cerebral ischemia and hypoxia.[5,8-10] It accomplishes these positive results largely by enhancing the oxygen use and increasing the cellular uptake of glucose, thus restoring aerobic glycolysis.

More specifically, GBE improves mitochondrial respiration, diminishes cerebral edema, improves membranal dynamics (including correction of ionic disturbances), stabilizes lysosomal membranes, and inhibits the action of proteolytic enzymes.[3] All these metabolic effects are in addition to GBE's ability to reestablish effective tissue perfusion. Most interesting is GBE's ability to normalize the circulation in the areas most affected by microembolization (small deposits of blood clots), namely, the hippocampus and striatum.[3]

GBE promotes an increased rate of nerve transmission, improved synthesis and turnover of cerebral neurotransmitters, and promotion of acetylcholine receptors in the hippocampus.[3] Further discussion of GBE's nervous tissue action occurs elsewhere in this chapter.

Vascular effects

The mechanisms of GBE's vascular effects have been investigated using a number of in vivo and in vitro techniques.[11] Isolated vessel techniques allow for separation of GBE's effects on different parts of the vascular system—e.g., arterial, arteriolar, microcirculatory, venular, and venous components—whereas in vivo studies provide information on the total circulatory phenomena (i.e., GBE's ability to increase the perfusion rate to various territories).

In general, GBE exerts its vascular effects primarily by affecting the cells that line the blood vessel and the tone of the smooth muscle cells of the vessel. Its vasodilating action is explained by direct stimulation of the release of endothelium-derived relaxing factor (EDRF) and prostacyclin. In addition, GBE inhibits enzymes in a way that leads to smooth muscle cell relaxation in the wall of the vessel.[11]

GBE also provides greater tone to the vein essential to the dynamic clearing of toxic metabolites that accumulate during low oxygen levels.[11] It is obvious that GBE produces a balanced action on the arterial and venous system, exerting tonic effects that are capable of restoring circulation in cases of vasomotor paralysis as well as relaxant effects in cases of vasomotor spasm. These effects are much more apparent in an ischemic vascular area than on a normally perfused area.[11]

Despite intense investigation, many of GBE's tonic effects on vascular components are still largely unexplained. It is truly remarkable that a substance can simultaneously combat the phenomena resulting from vascular spasm and with the same efficiency restore circulation to areas subject to vasomotor paralysis. The importance of this dual action is becoming more apparent in cerebral insufficiency because single direction drugs (i.e., vasodilators) can often aggravate the condition by dilating the healthy areas preferentially to the detriment of the hypoxic areas, thereby deflecting blood and oxygen away from the hypoxic area.

Platelet effects

GBE and isolated ginkgolides have profound effects on platelet function, including inhibition of platelet aggregation, adhesion, and degranulation.[3] These effects appear to be a result of direct membranal and antioxidant effects, increased synthesis of prostacyclin, inhibition of the enzyme phosphodiesterase, and antagonism of platelet activating factor.

As mentioned, GBE exerts membrane-stabilizing and free radical scavenging effects. Platelet membranes are quite sensitive to free radical damage, which then leads to hyperaggregation. Therefore, by stabilizing the platelet's membranes and scavenging damaging free radicals, GBE can greatly reduce platelet aggregation.

GBE also stimulates the synthesis of prostacyclin, the natural antiaggregatory prostaglandin synthesized by the vascular endothelium, the cells that line the inside of the vessel. This effect is in stark contrast to aspirin, which, although able to effectively reduce platelet aggregation, has a negative effect on prostacyclin synthesis.

GBE and the ginkgolides have been shown to be potent inhibitors of platelet activating factor (PAF-acether), ginkgolide B>A>C.[3,12-14] PAF-acether is a mediator derived from numerous cells and is a potent stimulator of platelet aggregation and degranulation. It is also involved in many inflammatory and allergic processes, including neutrophil activation, increasing vascular permeability, smooth muscle contraction including bronchoconstriction, and reduction in coronary blood flow.

GBE and ginkgolides compete with PAF-acether for binding cites. They also inhibit the various events induced by PAF-acether, including calcium influx and phospholipase activation.[3,12-14] These actions may be responsible for many of the clinical effects of GBE.

*GBE in cerebral vascular insufficiency
and impaired cerebral performance*

Cerebral vascular insufficiency is an extremely common condition in developed countries because of the high prevalence of atherosclerosis. In several studies (see Table 1), GBE has displayed a statistically significant regression of the major symptoms of cerebral vascular insufficiency and impaired cerebral performance. These symptoms include short-term memory loss, vertigo, headache, ringing in the ears, lack of vigilance ("get up and go"), and depression. The significant regression of these symptoms offered by GBE suggests that vascular insufficiency may indeed be the major causative factor that accounts for these so-called age-related cerebral disorders (as opposed to a true degenerative process).

It appears that *G. biloba* extract, by increasing cerebral blood flow, results in an increase in oxygen and glucose utilization, offers relief of these presumed side effects of aging, and may offer significant protection against the development of these symptoms. Furthermore, *G. biloba*'s antiaggregatory effect on platelets offers additional protection against a stroke. This effect has been supported in a clinical study in poststroke patients, which demonstrated that GBE improved blood and plasma viscosity.[37]

In addition to improving blood supply to the brain, *G. biloba* extract also increases the rate at which information is transmitted at the nerve cell level. This effect has been demonstrated in experimental and clinical studies.[25,26,38,39] In Hindmarch and Subhan's double-blind study, the time of reaction in healthy young women performing a memory test was improved significantly after GBE was administered.[38]

In another double-blind clinical study, *G. biloba* extract was shown to induce in elderly patients a restoration of vigilance toward normal levels and improved mental performace.[25] The findings at the behavioral level correlated with improvements in EEG (brain wave) tracings. The patients who had less favorable initial situation as measured in resting EEG activity displayed the greatest improvement. The study concluded that "chronic GBE medication has a positive effect in geriatric subjects with deterioration of mental performance and vigilance, and this effect is reflected at the behavioral level."

GBE should be taken consistently for at least 12 weeks in order to determine effectiveness. Although most people report benefits within a 2- to 3-week period, some individuals may take longer to respond. Warburton reviewed 20 carefully conducted studies involving a total of 770 patients observed for an average period of 4 months (ranging from 2 weeks to 1 year) and concluded: "It seems that the longer the treatment is continued, the more obvious and lasting the result. Even at the end of a year, it was found that improvement was continuing and adherence to the treatment was good.

Table 1 Studies demonstrating significant regression of the major symptoms of cerebral vascular insufficiency through the use of *G. biloba* extract

Principle author	Diagnosis	No. of patients	Age	Duration	Dosage	Compared to	Efficacy
Agnoli[17]	CCI	30	60	4 wk	120 mg	Placebo (n = 30)	76%
Arrigo[18]	CCI	80	40–80	7	120	Placebo (n = 40)	65%
Augustin[19]	Misc.	99	77	24	120	Placebo (n = 90)	44%
Bono[20]	CCI	14	65	5	120	Placebo (n = 14)	65%
	CCI	40	67	5	120	ED (n = 19)	90%
Boudouresques[21]	CCI, CVA	47	35–80	3	120		80%
Choussat[22]	CCI	48	65–95	8	360		60%
Dieli[23]	CCI	20	62	5	160	Placebo (n = 20)	80%
Eckmann[24]	CVA	25	60	4	120	Placebo (n = 20)	92%
Gessner[25]	Senescence	19	57–88	12	120	Placebo (n = 19) Nicergoline (n = 19)	69%
Hofferberth[26]	COS	36	53–69	8	120	Placebo (n = 18)	83%
Israel[27]	D	48	72	8	240		NS
Leroy[28]	CVA	27	78	8	120	Raubasine + ED (n = 24)	74%
Moreau[29]	CCI	30	84	12	120	Placebo (n = 30) ED (n = 30)	79%
Pidoux[30]	CCI	12	87	12	160	Placebo	85%
Sati[31]	CCI	20	47–86	2	35 (IV)		76%
Tea[33]	CVA	19	67	8	160		
Terasse[34]	Misc.	20	59–84	1–3	17.5 (IV)		55%
Vorberg[35]	CCI	112	55–94	52	120		68%
Wackenheim[36]	CCI	25	50	27	160		76%
	CCT	25	50	27	160		72%

CCI = chronic cerebral insufficiency; CCT = chronic cerebral trauma; COS = cerebral organic syndrome; CVA = cerebral vascular accidents; D = dementia; ED = ergot derivatives

At least eight days are necessary before the first clinical effects are manifested."[16]

GBE in Alzheimer's disease

G. biloba extract is showing great benefit in many cases of senility, including Alzheimer's disease.[16,23,29,40] In addition to GBE's ability to increase the functional capacity of the brain via the mechanisms described, it also has been shown to address many of the other major elements of Alzheimer's disease. (Studies show that GBE normalizes the muscarinic acetylcholine receptors in the hippocampus in aged animals and increases cholinergic transmission.[41])

Although preliminary studies in established Alzheimer's patients are quite promising,[40] at this time it appears that GBE can only help delay mental deterioration in the early stages of Alzheimer's disease, which may help to enable the patient to maintain a normal life and escape institutionalization. If the mental deficit is due to vascular insufficiency or depression and not to Alzheimer's disease, GBE will usually be effective in reversing the deficit.[16]

GBE in tinnitus

GBE has demonstrated favorable improvements in patients suffering from tinnitus (ringing in the ears) in two double-blind clinical studies.[42,43] In Meyer's study, GBE improved the condition regardless of prognostic factor, whereas Sprenger reported the complete abolition of tinnitus in 12 of 33 patients and improvement in 5 additional patients.

GBE in cochlear deafness

Lack of oxygen supply is the usual causative factor in acute cochlear deafness. GBE was shown to improve recovery in cases of acute cochlear deafness due to idiopathic sudden deafness or deafness caused by sound trauma or barotrauma.[44]

GBE in senile macular degeneration and diabetic retinopathy

GBE appears to address the disease process of senile macular degeneration quite effectively. In a small double-blind study, GBE demonstrated a statistically significant improvement in long-distance visual acuity.[45]

GBE has demonstrated impressive protective effects against free radical damage to the retina in experimental studies.[3,6,46,47] Furthermore, this extract has been shown to prevent diabetic retinopathy in chemically induced diabetic rats, which suggests that it may have a protective effect in human diabetics.[47]

GBE in peripheral arterial insufficiency

The primary lesion of atherosclerosis is the intimal plaque, which progressively narrows and ultimately blocks the artery, resulting in a decreased blood supply to the cells. A reduction in blood flow to an area induces a hypoxic event, which increases the production of toxic metabolites and cellular free radicals. These free radicals accumulate during reoxygenation and react with the cell membrane. This reaction commonly occurs in the leg. The result is a painful cramp (known as intermittent claudication).

GBE's free radical scavenging effect, combined with its vascular effects and its ability to increase metabolic processes during decreased blood supply, suggest that it may have clinical efficacy in cases of obliterative arterial disease and other causes of arterial insufficiency. Double-blind randomized clinical trials of *G. biloba* extract versus a placebo compared two parallel groups of patients with peripheral arterial insufficiency of the leg. In these trials, *G. biloba* extract was shown to be quite active and superior to the placebo.[48,49,50] Not only were measurements of pain-free walking distance and maximum walking distance dramatically increased, but plethysmographic and Doppler ultrasound measurements after exercise were also increased. These effects reflect increased blood flow through the affected limb.

The significance of these findings is great. Muscular rehabilitation and the elimination of risk factors (smoking, weight reduction, etc.) is the basis of medical treatment of patients with peripheral arterial insufficiency. However, the beneficial effects of such therapy on the walking tolerance has not been shown to be related to an improved perfusion of the limb, and results are limited over time. Therefore, the muscular rehabilitation and elimination of risk factors is not satisfactory alone. The fact that *G. biloba* extract improved limb blood flow and walking tolerance in studies that followed strict methodology and that had sufficient patients for reliable evaluation indicates that *G. biloba* extract should be the treatment of choice in peripheral arterial insufficiency.[51] This general disorder includes other peripheral vascular disorders such as diabetic peripheral vascular disease, Raynaud's syndrome, acrocyanosis, and postphlebitis syndrome.

GBE in erectile dysfunction

A preliminary clinical study indicated that GBE may be effective in impotency caused by arterial insufficiency.[52] The study included 60 patients with proven arterial erectile dysfunction who had not reacted to papaverine injections of up to 50 mg. These patients were treated with *Ginkgo biloba* extract in a dose of 60 mg/day for 12–18 months. The penile arterial blood flow was reevaluated by duplex sonography every 4 weeks.

The first signs of improved blood supply were seen after 6–8 weeks; after 6 months' therapy, 50% of the patients had regained potency, and in 20% a new trial of papaverine injection was then successful; 25% of the patients showed an improved arterial inflow, but papaverine was still not successful. The remaining 5% were unchanged.

The improvement of the arterial inflow is assumed to be the result of the known direct effect of *G. biloba* extract on endothelial cells, which enhances blood flow of both arteries and veins without any change in systemic blood pressure.

According to the results in this first open clinical trial, GBE appears very effective in the treatment of arterial erectile dysfunction. It reduces the need for intracavernosal drug injection and enhances arterial perfusion when using intracavernosal injection of papaverine or similar drugs. It must be noted again that ginkgo's effects are more apparent with long-term therapy.

GBE in idiopathic cyclic edema

Idiopathic cyclic edema is a frequent and often unrecognized condition in young women and is characterized by a water and sodium retention with secondary hyperaldosterism due to capillary hyperpermeability during the luteal phase of the menstrual cycle. GBE has demonstrated effective treatment for orthostatic idiopathic edema.[53]

Future applications of GBE

Experimental studies as well as some preliminary clinical evidence indicate that GBE may be of benefit as a vasodilator in cases of angina;[54] as an inotropic agent in congestive heart failure;[55] an antiallergy agent in asthma, urticaria (hives), and migraine;[12,56] in treating acute respiratory distress syndrome;[12,56] and as a mood-elevating substance in relieving depression.[57] Its action on PAF-acether may also make it useful for a great number of other applications, including various types of shock, thrombosis, graft protection during organ transplantation, multiple sclerosis, and thermal injury.[12-14]

Summary

G. biloba extract offers effective treatment for the signs and symptoms of arterial insufficiency. This has been confirmed by clinical studies in cases of cerebral arterial insufficiency and peripheral arterial insufficiency. GBE may lessen many common complaints of the geriatric population, such as senility, dizziness, ringing in the ears, depression, short-term memory loss, and intermittent claudication.

G. biloba extract may also improve mental functions and hearing loss in elderly patients by improving neural transmission. *G. biloba* extract may offer significant protective action against the development of Alzheimer's disease, hearing loss, and strokes.

Future clinical studies may indicate that GBE is of benefit as a vasodilator in cases of angina, as an inotropic agent in congestive heart failure, as a relaxant for smooth muscle, as an antiallergy agent in asthma and migraine, and as a mood-elevating substance in relieving depression.

Dosage

Most of the clinical research on *G. biloba* has used a standardized extract, containing 24% ginkgo heterosides (flavoglycosides), at a dose of 40 mg three times a day. It is difficult to devise a dosage schedule using other forms of ginkgo because of extreme variation in the content of active compounds in dried leaf and crude extracts. Whatever form of ginkgo is used, it appears to be essential that it be standardized for content and activity. If by chance a standard 1:5 tincture were obtained from the highest possible flavonoid content of crude ginkgo leaf, it would require 1 oz of the tincture per day to approach the equivalent dosage level of the standardized extract.[2]

Toxicology

There have not been any reports of significant adverse reactions to GBE at the prescribed dose. Mild adverse reactions, although quite rare, have been reported and include gastrointestinal upset and headache. Physicians in the United States using simple 8:1 extracts report a much higher incidence of side effects, presumably as a result of the presence of ginkgo constituents usually removed or altered by the standard extraction process.[2]

In contrast to the tolerance of the leaf, contact with or ingestion of the fruit pulp has produced severe allergic reactions.[58] Contact with the fruit pulp causes erythema and edema, with the rapid formation of vesicles accompanied by severe itching, similar to an allergic reaction to the sumacs (poison ivy and poison oak), which suggests a cross-reactivity between *G. biloba* fruit and the sumac group. Ingestion of as little as two pieces of fruit pulp has been reported to cause perioral erythema, rectal burning, and tenesmus.

References

1. Drieu K: Preparation and definition of Ginkgo biloba extract. In: Rokan (Ginkgo Biloba) - Recent Results in Pharmacology and Clinic. Funfgeld EW (ed). Springer-Verlag, New York, NY 1988, pp32-6
2. Bergner P: Ginkgo biloba. Medical Herbalism 2:1,5,6, 1990
3. Clostre F: From the body to the cellular membranes: The different levels of pharmacological action of Ginkgo biloba extract. In: Rokan (Ginkgo Biloba) - Recent Results in Pharmacology and Clinic. Funfgeld EW (ed). Springer-Verlag, New York, NY 1988, pp180-98
4. Schaffler VK and Reeh PW: Double-blind study of the hypoxia-protective effect of a standardized Ginkgo bilobae preparation after repeated administration in healthy volunteers. Arzneim-Forsch 35:1283-6, 1985
5. Chatterjee SS and Gabard B: Studies on the mechanism of action of an extract of Ginkgo biloba, a drug for the treatment of ischemic vascular diseases. Naunyn-Schmiedeberg's Arch Pharmacol 320:R52, 1982

6. Pincemail J and Deby C: The antiradical properties of Ginkgo biloba extract. In: Rokan (Ginkgo Biloba) - Recent Results in Pharmacology and Clinic. Funfgeld EW (ed). Springer-Verlag, New York, NY 1988, pp71-82

7. Etienne A, Hecquet F, Clostre F and DeFeudis FV: Comparison des effets d'un extrait de Ginkgo biloba et de la chlorpromazine sur la fragilite osmotique, in vitro, d'erythrocytes de rat. J Pharmacol 13:291-8, 1982

8. Le Poncin, Lafitte M, Rapin J, and Rapin JR: Effect of Ginkgo biloba on changes induced by quantitative cerebral microembolization in rats. Archs Int Pharmacodyn Ther 243:236-44, 1980

9. Karcher L, Zagerman P and Krieglstein J: Effect of an extract of Ginkgo biloba on rat brain energy metabolism in hypoxia. Naunyn-Schmiedeberg's Arch Pharmacol 327:31-5, 1984

10. Spinnewyn B, Blavet N and Clostre F: Effects of Ginkgo biloba extract on a cerebral ischemia model in gerbils. In: Rokan (Ginkgo Biloba) - Recent Results in Pharmacology and Clinic. Funfgeld EW (ed). Springer-Verlag, New York, NY 1988, pp143-52

11. Auguet M, Delaflotte S, Hellegouarch A and Clostre F: THe pharmacological bases for the vascular impact of ginkgo biloba extract. In: Rokan (Ginkgo Biloba) - Recent Results in Pharmacology and Clinic. Funfgeld EW (ed). Springer-Verlag, New York, NY 1988, pp169-79

12. Braquet P: Proofs of involvement of PAF-acether in various immune disorders using BN 52021 (Ginkgolide B): A powerful PAF-acether antagonist from Ginkgo biloba L. Adv Prost Thromb Leuko Res 16:179-98, 1986

13. Bourgain RH, Andries R and Braquet P: Effect of ginkgolide PAF-acether antagonists on arterial thrombosis. Adv Prost Thromb Leuko Res 17:815-7, 1987

14. Lamant V, Mauco G, Braquet P, et al: Inhibition of the metabolism of platelet activating factor (PAF-acether) by three specific antagonists from Ginkgo biloba. Biochemical Pharmacol 36:2749-52, 1987

15. Moreau JP, Eck CR, McCabe J and Skinner S: Absorption, distribution, and excretion of tagged Ginkgo biloba leaf extract in the rat. In: Rokan (Ginkgo Biloba) - Recent Results in Pharmacology and Clinic. Funfgeld EW (ed). Springer-Verlag, New York, NY 1988, pp37-45

16. Warburton DM: Clinical psychopharmacology of Ginkgo biloba extract. In: Rokan (Ginkgo Biloba) - Recent Results in Pharmacology and Clinic. Funfgeld EW (ed). Springer-Verlag, New York, NY 1988, pp327-45

17. Agnoli A: Clinical and psychometric aspects of the therapeutic effects of GBE. In: Effects of GBE and Organic Cerebral Impairment. Agnoli A and Rapin J (eds). John Libbey, London, 1985

18. Arrigo A and Cattaneo S: Clinical and psychometric evaluation of Ginkgo biloba extract in chronical cerebro-vascular diseases. In: Effects of GBE and Organic Cerebral Impairment. Agnoli A and Rapin J (eds). John Libbey, London, 1985

19. Augustin P: Le Tanakan en geriatrie; Etude clinique et psychometrique chez 189 malades d'hospice. Psychologie Medicale 8:123-30, 1976

20. Bono Y and Mouren P: L'insuffisance circulatoire cerebrale et son traitment par l'extrait de GInkgo biloba. Medit Med 3:59-62, 1975

21. Boudouresques G, Vigouroux R and Boudouresques J: Interet et place de l'extrait de Ginkgo biloba en pathologie vasculaire cerebrale. Med Pract 598:75-8, 1975

22. Choussat H, Beloussoff T, Dartenun JY and Emeriau JP: Essai clinique d'un extrait vegetal concentre en geriatrie. Geriatrie 2:370-5, 1977

23. Dieli G, La Mantia V, Saetta M and Costanzo E: Studio clinico in doppio cieco del Tanakan nell'insufficienza cerebrale cronica. Il Lavoro Neuropshiatrico 68:3, 1981

24. Eckmann VF and Schlag H: Kontrollierte doppelblind-studie zum wirksamkeitsnachweis von Tebonin forte bei patienten mit zerebrovakularer insuffizienz. Fortschr Med 31:1474-8, 1982

25. Gebner B, Voelp A and Klasser M: Study of the long-term action of a Ginkgo biloba extract on vigilance and mental performance as determined by means of quantitative pharmaco-EEG and psychometric measurements. Arzneim Forsch 35:1459-65, 1985

26. Hofferberth B: Effect of Ginkgo biloba extract on neurophysiological and psychometric measurment in patients with cerebro-organic syndrome - A double-blind study versus placebo. Arzneim Forsch 39:918-22, 1989

27. Leroy H, Saluan P, Chovelon R and Bouilloux E: Approche clinique et psychometrique en geriatrie. Methodes d'etudes et choix d'une therapeutique. Vie Medicale 19:2513-9, 1978

28. Moreau P: Un nouveau stimulant circulatoire cerebral. Nouv Presse Med 4:2401-2, 1975

29. Israel L, Ohlman T, Delomier Y and Hugonot R: Etude psychometrique de l'activite d'un extrait vegetal au cours des etats d'involution senile. Lyon Medit Medical 13:1197-9, 1977

30. Pidoux B, Bastien C and Niddam S: Clinical and quantitative EEG double-blind study of GBE. J Cerebral Blood Flow Metabol 3:5556-7, 1983

31. Safi N and Galley P: Tanakan et cerveau senile. Etude radiocicrculographique. Bordeaux Medical 10:171-6, 1977

32. Taillandier J, Ammar A, Rabourdin JP, et al: Ginkgo biloba extract in the treatment of cerebral disorders due to aging - Longitudinal, multicenter, double-blind study versus placebo. In: Rokan (Ginkgo Biloba) - Recent Results in Pharmacology and Clinic. Funfgeld EW (ed). Springer-Verlag, New York, NY 1988, pp291-301

33. Tea S, Celsis P, Clanet M and Marc-Vergnes JP: Effets cliques, hemodynamiques et metabloiques de l'extrait de Ginkgo biloba en pathologie vasculaire cerebrale. Gazz Med France 86:4149-52, 1979

34. Terasse J and Morin B: Experimentaion du Tanakan par voie parenterale. Lyon Medical 245:841-2, 1976

35. Vorberg G: Ginkgo biloba extract (GBE): A long-term study of chronic cerebral insufficiency in geriatric patients. Clinical Trials Journal 22:149-57, 1985

36. Wackenheim A: Essai clinique du Tanakan dans le syndrome fonctionnel des traumatises du crane et l'insuffisance vasculaire cerebrale. Med du Nord et de l'Est 1:73-8, 1977

37. Anadere I, Chmiel H and Witte S: Hemorrheological findings in patients with completed stroke and the influence of GInkgo biloba extract. Clin Hemorheo 4:411-20, 1985

38. Hindmarch I and Subhan Z: The psychopharmacological effects of Ginkgo biloba extract in normal healthy volunteers. Int J Clin Pharmacol Res 4:89-93, 1984

39. Pidoux B: Effects of Ginkgo biloba extract on cerebral functional activity - Results of clincal and experimental studies. In: Rokan (Ginkgo Biloba) - Recent Results in Pharmacology and Clinic. Funfgeld EW (ed). Springer-Verlag, New York, NY 1988, pp314-20

40. Funfgeld EW: A natural and broad spectrum nootropic substance for treatment of SDAT - the Ginkgo biloba extract. In: Alzheimer's Disease and Related Disorders. Iqbal K, Sisniewski HM and Winblad B (eds). Alan Liss, New York, NY, 1989, pp1247-60

41. Allard M: Treatment of old age disorders with Ginkgo biloba extract - From pharmacology to clinic. In: Rokan (Ginkgo Biloba) - Recent Results in Pharmacology and Clinic. Funfgeld EW (ed). Springer-Verlag, New York, NY 1988, pp201-11

42. Meyer B: A multicenter randomized double-blind study of Ginkgo biloba extract versus placebo in the treatment of tinnitus. In: Rokan (Ginkgo Biloba) - Recent Results in Pharmacology and Clinic. Funfgeld EW (ed). Springer-Verlag, New York, NY 1988, pp245-50

43. Sprenger FH: Gute therapie ergebnissemit Ginkgo biloba. Arztlich Praxis 12:938-40, 1986

44. Dubreuil C: Therapeutic trial in acute cochlear deafness - Comparative study with Ginkgo biloba extract and nicergoline. In: Rokan (Ginkgo Biloba) - Recent Results in Pharmacology and Clinic. Funfgeld EW (ed). Springer-Verlag, New York, NY 1988, pp237-44

45. Lebuisson DA, Leroy L and Rigal G: Treatment of senile macular degeneration with Ginkgo biloba extract. A preliminary double-blind, drug versus placebo study. In: Rokan (Ginkgo Biloba) - Recent Results in Pharmacology and Clinic. Funfgeld EW (ed). Springer-Verlag, New York, NY 1988, pp231-6

46. Doly M and Braquet P: Effet des radicaux libres oxygenes sur l'activite electrophysiologique de la retine isolee de rat. J Fr Ophtalmol 8:273-7, 1985

47. Doly M, Droy-Lefaix MT, Bonhomme B, and Braquet P: Effectof Ginkgo biloba extract on the electrophysiology of the isolated diabetic rat retina. In: Rokan (Ginkgo Biloba) - Recent Results in Pharmacology and Clinic. Funfgeld EW (ed). Springer-Verlag, New York, NY 1988, pp83-90

48. Bauer U: 6-Month double-blind randomized clinical trial of Ginkgo biloba extract versus placebo in two parallel groups in patients suffering from peripheral arterial insufficiency. Arzneim-Forsch 34:716-21, 1984

49. Courbier R, Jausseran JM and Reggi M: Etude a double insu coissee du Tanakan dans les arteriopathies des membres inferieurs. Medit Med 126:61-4, 1977

50. Rudofsky VG: The effect of Ginkgo biloba extract in cases of arterial occlusive disease - A randomized placebo controlled double-blind cross-over study. Fortschr Med 105:397-400, 1987

51. Bauer U: Ginkgo biloba extract in the treatment of arteriopathy of the lower limbs - sixty five week study. In: Rokan (Ginkgo Biloba) - Recent Results in Pharmacology and Clinic. Funfgeld EW (ed). Springer-Verlag, New York, NY 1988, pp212-20

52. Sikora R, Sohn M, Deutz FJ, et al: Ginkgo biloba extract in the therapy of erectile dysfunction. Journal of Urology 141:188A, 1989

53. Lagrue G, Behar A, Kazandjian M and Rahbar K: Idiopathic cyclic edema - Role of capillary hyperpermeability and its correction by Ginkgo biloba extract. In: Rokan (Ginkgo Biloba) - Recent Results in Pharmacology and Clinic. Funfgeld EW (ed). Springer-Verlag, New York, NY 1988, pp221-7

54. Guillon JM, Rochette L and Baranes J: Effects of Ginkgo biloba extract on two models of experimental myocardial ischemia. In: Rokan (Ginkgo Biloba) - Recent Results in Pharmacology and Clinic. Funfgeld EW (ed). Springer-Verlag, New York, NY 1988, pp153-61

55. Beretz A, Joly M, Stoclet JC, and Anton R: Inhibition of 3',5'-AMP phosphodiesterase by biflavonoids and xanthones. Planta Medica 36:193-5, 1979

56. Puglisi L, Salvadori S, Gabrielli G and Pasargiklian R: Pharmacology of natural compounds.I. Smooth

muscle relaxant activity induced by a Ginkgo biloba L. extract on guinea-pig trachea. Pharmacol Res Commun 20:573-89, 1988

57. Brunello N, Racagni G, Clostre F, et al: Effects of an extract of Ginkgo biloba on noradrenergic systems of rat cerebral cortex. Pharmacological Research Commun 17:1063-72, 1985

58. Becker LE and Skipworth GB: Ginkgo-tree dermatitis, stomatitis, and proctitis. JAMA 231:1162-3, 1975

17

Gugulipid

Key uses of gugulipid:

- Elevated cholesterol and triglyceride levels
- Atherosclerosis
- Hypothyroidism

General description

Gugulipid is the standardized extract of the oleoresin of *Commiphora mukul* (mukul myrrh tree), an Indian medicinal tree.

Chemical composition

The active components of gugulipid are two compounds, Z-guggulsterone and E-guggulsterone. For best results, gugulipid should be standardized to contain a minimum of 4% guggulsterone. Other components of gugulipid include various diterpenes, sterols, steroids, esters, and fatty alcohols.[1]

Pharmacology

Gugulipid is an effective lipid-lowering agent.[1-4] It lowers both cholesterol and triglyceride levels. Gugulipid's effect on cholesterol is extremely beneficial because it lowers LDL-cholesterol while simultaneously elevating HDL-cholesterol. (HDL-cholesterol has been shown to offer protection against heart disease due to atherosclerosis.)

Studies have shown that gugulipid prevents the formation of atherosclerosis and aids in the regression of pre-existing atherosclerotic plaques. This extract also appears to prevent heart damage by free radicals as well as to improve the metabolism of the heart. Gugulipid has a mild effect in inhibiting platelets from aggregating.[1]

An extremely interesting action of guggulsterone is its ability to stimulate thyroid function.[5] This thyroid-stimulating effect may be responsible for some of this extract's lipid-lowering activity.

Several clinical studies have confirmed that gugulipid has an ability to lower both cholesterol and triglyceride levels.[1-4] Typically, cholesterol levels will drop 14–27% in a 4- to 12-week period, and triglyceride levels will drop 22–30%.

The effect of gugulipid on serum cholesterol and triglycerides is comparable to that of other lipid-lowering drugs. Clofibrate, niacin, and cholestyramine lower cholesterol levels 6–12%, 10–17% and 20–27%, respectively, but are associated with some degree of toxicity. In contrast, gugulipid has no side effects. The mechanism of action for gugulipid cholesterol-lowering action is its ability to increase the liver's metabolism of LDL-cholesterol—i.e., guggulsterone increases the uptake of LDL-cholesterol from the blood by the liver.[6]

Summary

Gugulipid is an effective agent in protecting against (and in treating) atherosclerotic disease. Its ability to lower cholesterol and triglycerides makes it valuable for related conditions.

Dosage

The dosage of gugulipid is based on its guggulsterone content. Clinical studies have demonstrated that the equivalent of 25 mg of guggulsterone three times a day is an effective treatment for elevated cholesterol levels, elevated triglyceride levels, or both. For a 4% guggulsterone content extract, the most effective dose is approximately 500–600 mg three times a day.

Toxicology

Safety studies with rats, rabbits, and monkeys have demonstrated that gugulipid is nontoxic.[1] It does not have any embryotoxic or fetotoxic effects. It is therefore considered safe to use during pregnancy.

References

1. Gugulipid. Drugs of the Future 13:618-9, 1988
2. Agarwal RC, Singh SP, Saran RK, et al: Clinical trial of gugulipid a new hypolipidemic agent of plant origin in primary hyperlipidemia. Ind J Med Res 84:626-34, 1986
3. Nityanand S, Srivastava JS and Asthana OP: Clinical trials with gugulipid, a new hypolipidaemic agent. J Assoc Phys India 37:321-8, 1989
4. Kuppurajan K, Rajagopalan SS, Koteswara RT and Sitaraman R: Effect of gugglu on serum lipids in obese hypercholesterolemic and hyperlipidemic cases. J Assoc Phys India 26:367-71, 1978
5. Tripathi YB, Tripathi P, Malhorta P and Tripathi SN: Thyroid stimulatory action of (Z)-gugulsterone: mechanism of action. Planta Medica 54:271-7, 1988
6. Singh V, Kaul S, Chander R and Kapoor NK: Stimulation of low density lipoprotein receptor activity in liver membrane of guggulsterone treated rats. Pharmacol Res 22:37-44, 1990

SECTION VI

*Herbs for the lungs
and respiratory system*

The lungs are paired, cone-shaped organs that lie in the chest cavity. Each day we take in (and let out) about 20,000 breaths to replenish our bodies with oxygen and eliminate carbon dioxide. Over 10,000,000 ml of air pass into the lungs each day. In addition to containing oxygen and other gases, air is composed of dirt, dust, pollen, microbes, cigarette smoke, and other pollutants. Often, the lungs are damaged or become sensitive to pollutants. Two herbs that help restore health and vitality to the lungs are lobelia and ephedra. This section highlights these two effective herbs.

18

Lobelia

(LOBELIA INFLATA)

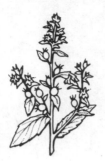

Key uses of lobelia:

- Smoking deterrent
- Asthma
- Bronchitis
- Pneumonia

General description

Lobelia, or Indian tobacco, is an indigenous North American annual or biennial plant that has an erect, angular, hairy stem. The stem contains a milky sap and grows 6 in. to 3 ft in height. Numerous small, two-lipped, blue flowers grow in spikelike racemes from July to November.

Chemical composition

Lobelia contains about 0.48% pyridine (piperidine) alkaloids composed mainly of lobeline, with lesser amounts of lobelanine, lobelanidine, and other alkaloids. Other constituents include resin, gum, lipids, and chelidonic acid.[1-3]

History and folk use

Lobelia was used extensively by Thomsonians (see the Introduction) as an emetic, a diaphoretic, an expectorant, a sedative, an antispasmodic, and an antiasthmatic. It has been used to treat asthma, whooping cough, bruises, sprains, ringworm, insect bites, poison ivy symptoms, and many other conditions. Thomson stated, "There is no vegetable which the earth produces more harmless in its effect on the human system, and none more powerful in removing disease and promoting health than lobelia."[4] Lobelia has also been used as a stop-smoking aid.

Pharmacology

Lobelia's pharmacology centers around its lobeline content. Lobeline has many of the same pharmacological actions as nicotine but is generally regarded as being less potent.[5,6] Lobeline is often used as a smoking deterrent to lessen nicotine withdrawal.[1,2]

Gastrointestinal effects

The emetic action of lobeline is mediated by its stimulation of the vomiting center at the base of the brain, the area postrema of the medulla oblongata, which is outside the blood-brain barrier.[7]

Respiratory effects

Lobelia is a very effective expectorant. (Expectorants modify the quality and quantity of the secretions of the respiratory tract resulting in the expulsion of secretions and an improvement in respiratory tract function.) Lobelia is used as an expectorant primarily in such conditions as pneumonia, asthma, and bronchitis. It appears that its major actions are a result of stimulating the adrenal gland to release hormones that cause the bronchial muscles to relax.[8,9]

Although lobelia may be effective when used alone in the treatment of asthma, it has traditionally been used in combination with other herbs.[10] Typically, it is combined with *Capsicum frutescens* (cayenne pepper) and *Symplocarpus foetidus* (skunk cabbage).

Summary

Many of lobelia's effects are related to its lobeline content. Lobelia is particularly useful as an expectorant in respiratory tract conditions like asthma, pneumonia, and bronchitis. Lobelia can also be used as a smoking deterrent.

Dosage

Dosages of three times a day are as follows:

- Dried herb or as infusion (tea)—0.5–1 g
- Tincture (1:5)—4–6 ml (1–1½ tsp)
- Fluid extract (1:1)—0.5–1 ml (⅛–¼ tsp)
- Solid extract (dried, powdered), of 1% lobeline content—200 mg

Toxicology

Ingestion of toxic levels of lobelia usually results in vomiting, thereby lessening the likelihood of a fatal outcome.[4] Toxic symptoms, which resemble nicotine poisoning, include nausea, salivation, diarrhea, disturbed hearing and vision, mental confusion, and marked weakness. Faintness and prostration ensue; blood pressure falls; the pulse becomes weak, rapid, and irregular; breathing is difficult; and collapse occurs followed by convulsions. Death may result from respiratory failure.[5] The antidote in acute poisoning is 2 mg of atropine given subcutaneously.[11]

References

1. Leung A: Encyclopedia of Common Natural Ingredients Used in Food, Drugs, and Cosmetics. John Wiley & Sons, New York, NY, 1980. pp220-3
2. Tyler V, Brady L, and Robbers J: Pharmacognosy, 8th ed. Lea & Febiger, Philadelphia, Pa, 1981. pp68-70
3. Merck Index, 10th ed. Merck & Co, Rahway, NJ, 1983. p4374
4. Christopher J: School of Natural Healing. BiWorld Publishers, Provo, Utah, 1976. pp358-367
5. Gilman A, Goodman L, and Gilman A: The Pharmacological Basis of Therapeutics. MacMillan Publ, New York, NY, 1980. pp212-4
6. Mansuri S, Kelkar V, and Jindal M: Some pharmacological characteristics of ganglionic activity of lobeline. Arzneim Forsch 23:1271-5, 1973
7. Laffan R and Borison H: Emetic action of nicotine and lobeline. J Pharmacol Exp Ther 121:468-476, 1957
8. Halmagyi D, Kovacs A, and Neumann P: Adrenocortical pathway of lobeline protection in some forms of experimental lung edema of the rat. Dis Chest 33:285-296, 1958
9. Cambar P, Shore S and Aviado D: Bronchopulmonary and gastrointestinal effects of lobeline. Arch Int Pharmacodyn 177:1-27, 1969
10. Mitchell W: Naturopathic Applications of the Botanical Remedies. Seattle, Wa, 1983
11. Dreisbach RH: Handbook of Poisoning. Lange Med Publ, Los Altos, Ca, 1983. p553

19

Ephedra

(EPHEDRA SINICA)

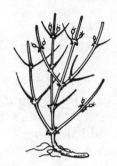

Key uses of ephedra:

- Asthma
- Hay fever
- Common cold
- Weight-loss aid

General description

Ephedra species are erect, branching shrubs found in desert or arid regions throughout the world. *Ephedra sinica* (Chinese ephedra or Ma Haung) is found in Asia; *E. distacha* (European ephedra) is found in Europe; *E. trifurca* or *E. viridis* (desert tea), *E. nevadensis* (Mormon tea), and *E. americana* (American ephedra) are found in North America; and *E. gerardiana* (Pakistani ephedra) is found primarily in India and Pakistan. The 1.5–4-ft shrubs typically grow on dry, rocky, or sandy slopes. The many slender, yellow-green branches of ephedra have two very small leaf scales at each node. The mature, double-seeded cones are visible in the fall.

Chemical composition

The chemical analysis of the stems and branches of *Ephedra* sp. has focused on the alkaloid content. In *E. sinica*, the total alkaloid content can be up to 3.3%, with 40–90% of this being ephedrine and the remaining alkaloids being primarily pseudoephedrine and nor-pseudoephedrine. In *E. gerardiana*, the alkaloid content usually varies from 0.8 to 1.4% and consists of about half ephedrine and half other alkaloids (pseudoephedrine, N-methyl-ephedrine, norephedrine, etc.). Mormon tea, or *E. nevadensis*, is reported to contain no ephedrine.[1,2]

History and folk use

The medicinal use of *E. sinica* in China dates from approximately 2800 B.C. *Ma Huang* refers to the stem and branch, and *Ma Huanggen* refers to the root and rhizome. Ma Huang was used primarily in the treatment of the common cold, asthma, hay fever, bronchitis, edema, arthritis, fever, hypotension, and urticaria.[1] Ma Huanggen is believed to produce effects opposite those of the stem and branches. Its use was limited to the treatment of profuse night sweating.[3]

Western medicine's interest in ephedra began in 1923, with the demonstration that the isolated alkaloid ephedrine possessed a number of pharmacological effects.[3] Ephedrine was synthesized in 1927. Since then, both ephedrine and pseudoephedrine have been used extensively in over-the-counter cold and allergy medications.[3]

Pharmacology

The pharmacology of ephedra centers around its ephedrine content. Ephedrine and pseudoephedrine have been extensively investigated and are widely used in prescription and over-the-counter medications for asthma, hay fever, and rhinitis.[3] In 1973, more than 20 million prescriptions written contained either of these alkaloids.

Ephedrine

Ephedrine's basic pharmacological action is similar to that of epinephrine (adrenaline), although ephedrine is much less active. Ephedrine also differs from epinephrine in its ability to be absorbed orally. It is active for a longer period of time, and it has a more pronounced effect on the brain and central nervous system (CNS). The CNS effects of ephedrine are similar to those of amphetamines; again, ephedrine's effects are much less potent.[3]

The cardiovascular effects of ephedrine are also similar to those of epinephrine—i.e., ephedrine increases blood pressure, cardiac output, and heart rate—but is much longer in duration (about 10 times). Like epinephrine, ephedrine will increase heart, brain, and muscle blood flow at the expense of kidney and intestinal blood flow.[3] Ephedrine relaxes the bronchial muscles, the muscles of the airways, and the muscles of the uterus.[3]

Pseudoephedrine

Pseudoephedrine exhibits similar bronchial muscle-relaxing activity to ephedrine, but it has weaker effects on the heart and CNS. Pseudoephedrine is often recommended over ephedrine in the treatment of chronic asthma because it has fewer side effects.[3]

Pseudoephedrine has also demonstrated significant anti-inflammatory effect in various experimental models.[4,5] Other ephedra alkaloids, including ephedrine, also exhibited anti-inflammatory activity but at much lower potency.

Ephedra and pseudoephedrine in asthma and hay fever

Ephedra and its alkaloids have proved to be effective bronchodilators for the treatment of mild to moderate asthma and hay fever.[3] The peak bronchodilation effect occurs in 1 hr and lasts about 5 hr after administration.

The therapeutic effect of ephedra will diminish if used over a long period of time due to weakening of the adrenal gland caused by ephedrine. It is therefore often necessary to use ephedra in combination with adrenal gland supportive herbs like licorice (*Glycyrrhiza glabra*) and *Panax ginseng*, as well as nutrients that support the adrenal glands, like vitamin C, magnesium, zinc, vitamin B_6, and pantothenic acid.

The old-time herbal treatment of asthma involves the use of ephedra in combination with herbal expectorants, such as licorice (*Glycyrrhiza glabra*), grindelia (*Grindelia camporum*), euphorbia (*Euphorbia hirta*), sundew (*Drosera rotundifolia*), and senega (*Polygala senega*).

Ephedra as a weight-loss aid

Studies with humans and laboratory animals have shown that ephedrine promotes weight loss.[6-10] Although ephedrine has an appetite-suppressing effect,[6] its main mechanism for promoting weight loss appears to be increasing the metabolic rate of adipose tissue.[7] Its weight-reducing effects are greatest in those individuals who have a low basal metabolic rate.

Although ephedrine is somewhat effective on its own as a weight-loss aid, it can be greatly enhanced when used in combination with caffeine and theophylline. These methylxanthines potentiate the action of ephedrine and other ephedra compounds.

In one animal study, when ephedrine was used alone it resulted in losses of 14% in body weight and 42% in body fat; when it was used in combination with caffeine or theophylline, there was a loss of 25% in body weight and 75% in body fat.[9] In contrast, when either caffeine or theophylline were used alone, there was no significant loss in body weight. The reason for the decrease in body weight is an increased metabolic rate and fat cell breakdown, promoted by ephedrine and enhanced by caffeine and theophylline.

It is recommended that green tea (*Camellia sinensis*) or extracts of *Cola* sp. be used for methylxanthine content rather than coffee. Coffee contains many roasted hydrocarbons that are known to be potent carcinogens. Researchers have suggested that it is not the caffeine content of coffee that is detrimental but the roasted hydrocarbons.[11]

Summary

Ephedra sp. may be used effectively to treat chronic asthma and hay fever as well as relieving common cold symptoms. Because it speeds metabolism, it is also an effective weight-loss aid. The alkaloid ephedrine is the primary active component in the herb *Ephedra* sp.

Dosage

The dosage of ephedra depends on its alkaloid content. The average total alkaloid content of *E. sinica* is 1–3%. For asthma and weight loss, the dose should have an ephedrine content of 12.5–25.0 mg and be taken two or three times a day. This would require a dose of 500–1,000 mg of the crude herb three times a day. Standardized preparations are preferred because they are more dependable for therapeutic activity. For example, *E. sinica* extracts are available that have a standardized alkaloid content of 10%. The dosage of a 10% alkaloid content extract would be 125–250 mg three times a day.

Toxicology

Ephedra can produce the same side effects that ephedrine can—i.e., increased blood pressure, increased heart rate, insomnia, and anxiety. The FDA advisory review panel on nonprescription drugs recommends that ephedrine not be taken by patients with heart disease, high blood pressure, thyroid disease, diabetes, or difficulty in urination due to enlargement of the prostate gland. In addition, ephedrine should not be used by patients on antihypertensives or antidepressants.

References

1. Chang HM and But PP: Pharmacology and Applications of Chinese Materia Medica, volume 2. World Scientific Publishing, Teaneck, NJ, 1987
2. Duke JA: Handbook of Medicinal Herbs. CRC Press, Boca Raton, FL 1985
3. Gilman AG, Goodman AS and Gilman A: The Pharmacologic Basis of Therapeutics. MacMillan Publishing, New York, NY 1980
4. Hikino H, Konno C, Takata H and Tamada M: Antiinflammatory principle of ephedra herbs. Chem Pharm Bull 28:2900-4, 1980
5. Kasahara Y, Hikino H, Tsuru S, Watanabe M and Ohuchi K: Antiinflammatory actions of ephedrines in acute inflammations. Planta Medica 54:325-31, 1985
6. Zarrindast MR, Hosseini-Nia and Farnoodi F: Anorectic effect of ephedrine. Gen Pharmacol 18:559-61, 1987
7. Astrup A, Madsen J, Holst JJ and Christensen NJ: The effect of chronic ephedrine treatment on substrate utilization, the sympathoadrenal activity, and expenditure during glucose-induced thermogenesis in man. Metabolism 35:260-5, 1986
8. Bailey CJ, Thornburn CC and Flatt PR: Effects of ephedrine and atenol on the development of obesity and diabetes in ob/ob mice. Gen Pharmac 17:243-6, 1986
9. Dulloo AG and Miller DS: The thermogenic properties of ephedrine/methylxanthine mixtures: animal studies. Am J Clin Nutr 43:388-94, 1986
10. Pasquali R, Cesari MP, Melchionda N, et al: Does ephedrine promote weight loss in low-energy-adapted obese women? Int J Obesity 11:163-8, 1985
11. Pozniak PC: The carcinogenicity of caffeine and coffee: A review. J Am Dietetic Assoc ADA 85:1127-33, 1985

SECTION VII

Herbs for urinary tract disorders

This section highlights two important herbs for the urinary tract. Saw palmetto is nature's answer to benign prostate enlargement. Uva ursi is an excellent urinary tract antiseptic that is useful in a wide range of urinary tract infections.

20

Saw palmetto

(SERENOA REPENS)

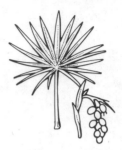

Key uses of saw palmetto:

- Benign prostate enlargement
- Decreased function of testes

General description

Serenoa repens (saw palmetto) is a small palm tree native to the Atlantic Coast of North America from South Carolina to Florida. The plant grows 6–10 ft high with a crown of large leaves. The berries of the plant are the components used for medicinal purposes. The deep red-brown to black berries are wrinkled, oblong, and 0.5–1 in. long with a diameter of 0.5 in.[1]

Chemical composition

Saw palmetto berries contain about 1.5% of an oil made of saturated and unsaturated fatty acids and sterols.[1] About 63% of the oil is composed of free fatty acids, including capric, caprylic, caproic, lauric, palmitic, and oleic acids. The remaining portion of the oil is composed of ethyl esters of these fatty acids and sterols, including beta-sitosterol and its glucoside. The lipid-soluble compounds are thought to be the major pharmacological components. Other components of the berries include carotenes, lipase, tannins, and sugars.

The purified fat-soluble extract that is used medicinally contains no less than 85% and no more than 95% fatty acids and sterols. This extract is made up predominantly of a complex mixture of saturated and unsaturated free fatty acids (approximately 85%), their methyl- and ethyl-esters (approximately 7%), long-chain alcohols in free and esterified form and various free and esterified sterol derivatives.

The free fatty acid compounds identified in this extract by gas chromatography and mass spectrometry include capronic acid (C_6), capric acid (C_8), caprylic acid (C_{10}), lauric acid (C_{12}), mirystic acid (C_{14}), isomirystic acid (C_{14}), palmitic acid (C_{16}), oleic acid ($C_{18:1}$), and stearic acid (C_{18}). Lauric and mirystic acid are the major fatty acids; they account for approximately 30% of the fatty acid content.

The identified alcohols include those with n-C_{22}, n-C_{23}, n-C_{24}, nC_{26}, nC_{28}, and nC_{30} chains, phytol, farnesol, and geranylgeraniol, in addition to high molecular weight unsaturated polyprenols.

The sterolic fraction is composed of beta-sitosterol, stigmasterol, cycloartenol, lupeol, lupenone, and 24-methylcycloartenol. Many of these sterols are esterified with the fatty acids of the extract.

History and folk use

Native Americans and, later, Eclectic physicians used saw palmetto in the treatment of genitourinary tract disturbances and as a tonic to support nutrients in the body. It was used in men to increase the function of the testicles and in women with disorders of the mammary glands. Many herbalists have regarded it has an aphrodisiac.[1]

Pharmacology

The standardized liposterolic (fat-soluble) saw palmetto berry extract has demonstrated numerous pharmacological effects in addition to nutritional qualities. Specifically, it has demonstrated antiandrogen and antiedema effects.[1-4] Saw palmetto polysaccharides have demonstrated immune-stimulating effects in vitro.[5]

Currently, the prime therapeutic application of *S. repens* berries (specifically, the fat-soluble extract) is in the treatment of a common disorder of the prostate gland, benign prostatic hyperplasia (BPH). Studies have indicated that 50–60% of men between the ages of 40 and 59 years have BPH. BPH is characterized by increased urinary frequency, nighttime awakening to empty the bladder, and reduced force and caliber of urination.

If BPH is left untreated, eventually the bladder outlet will be obstructed, resulting in the retention of urine in the blood (a condition known as uremia). For this reason, surgical intervention is often necessary. The annual overall cost of hospital care and surgery for benign prostatic hyperplasia in this country is over $1 billion.

BPH is thought to be caused by an accumulation of the male sex hormone testosterone in the prostate. Once within the prostate, testosterone is converted to an even more potent compound, dihydrotestosterone (DHT), which causes cells to multiply excessively and eventually causes the prostate to enlarge.

The liposterolic saw palmetto berry extract has been shown to prevent the conversion of testosterone to dihydrotestosterone as well as inhibit DHT's binding to cellular and nuclear receptor sites, thereby increasing the breakdown and excretion of DHT.[2,3] These effects are believed to be the reasons for the impressive clinical results obtained with the saw palmetto extract.[6-16]

The positive clinical results of the liposterolic extract of *Serenoa* on the major symptoms of BPH have been confirmed in several double-blind, placebo-controlled clinical trials.[6-16] (See Table 1.)

For example, Champault et al.'s double-blind placebo-controlled study of 110 outpatients suffering from BPH obtained impressive clinical results.[16] Nocturia (measured by number of times) decreased by over 45%, flow rate (ml/s) increased by over 50%, and residual urine content of the bladder (ml) decreased by 42% in the group receiving the *Serenoa* extract. In contrast, those on placebo did not significantly improve in nocturia or flow rate and actually worsened in residual urine content of the bladder.

Significant improvements were also noted in self-rating by the patients and global rating by the physician. Of the 50 subjects who completed the 30-day study and who had taken the liposterolic extract of *Serenoa*, physician's rating noted 14 had greatly improved, 31 had improved, and only 5 had remained unchanged or worsened. In contrast, no subjects in the placebo group had greatly improved, 16 showed some improvement, and 28 remained unchanged or worse.

Summary

The liposterolic extract of the berries of *S. repens* offers significant relief for the symptoms of benign prostatic hyperplasia. Furthermore, its pharmacology suggests it may be useful in the treatment of hirsutism and androgen excess in women.

Dosage

The dosage for the liposterolic extract of saw palmetto berries containing 85–95% fatty acids and sterols is 160 mg twice a day. To achieve a similar dose

Table 1 Clinical studies demonstrating the efficacy of *S. repens** in BPH

Authors	Type of study	Number of patients	Length of study	Results
Boccafoschi et al.l.	Double-blind, placebo-controlled	22	60 days	Significant difference for volume voided, maximum flow, mean flow, dysuria, nocturia
Cirillo et al.	Open	47	4 months	Significant difference for dysuria, nocturia, urine flow
Tripodi et al.	Open	40	30–90 days	Significant difference for dysuria, nocturia, volume of prostate, voiding rate, residual urine
Emili et al.	Double-blind, placebo-controlled	30	30 days	Significant difference for number of voidings, strangury, maximum and mean urine flow, residual urine
Greca et al.	Open	14	1–2 months	Significant difference for dysuria, perineal heaviness, nocturia, volume of urine per voiding, interval between two diurnal voidings, sensation of incomplete voiding
Duvia et al.	Controlled trial vs. *Pygeum africanum*	30	30 days	Significant difference for voiding rate
Tamca et al.	Double-blind, placebo-controlled	30	31–90 days	Significant difference for frequency, urine flow measurement
Cukier et al.	Double-blind, placebo-controlled	168	60–90 days	Significant difference for dysuria, frequency, residual urine
Crimi et al.	Open	32	4 weeks	Significant difference for dysuria, nocturia, volume of prostate, voiding rate
Champault et al.	Double-blind, placebo-controlled	110	28 days	Significant difference for dysuria, nocturia, flow measurement, residual urine

*Daily dosage 320 mg

using the crude berries would require a dose of at least 10 g twice a day. Dosages for fluid extracts and tinctures would result in extremely large quantities of alcohol and therefore cannot be recommended.

Toxicology

No significant side effects have been reported in the clinical trials of the saw palmetto berry extract or with saw palmetto berry ingestion.

References

1. Duke JA: Handbook of Medicinal Herbs. CRC Press, Boca Raton, Fl 1985. p118
2. Carilla E, Briley M, Fauran F, et al: Binding of Permixon, a new treatment for prostatic benign hyperplasia, to the cytosolic androgen receptor in the rat prostate. J Steroid Biochem 20:521-3, 1984
3. Sultan C, Terraza A, Devillier C, et al: Inhibition of androgen metabolism and binding by a liposterolic extract of "Serenoa repens B" in human foreskin fibroblasts. J Steroid Biochem 20:515-9, 1984
4. Tarayre JP, Delhon A, Lauressergues H, et al: Anti-edematous action of a hexane extract of the stone fruit of Serenoa repens Bartr. Ann Pharm Franc 41:559-70, 1983
5. Wagner H and Proksch A: Immunostimulatory drugs of fungi and higher plants. Econ Med Plant Res 1:113-53, 1985
6. Boccafoschi and Annoscia S: Comparison of Serenoa repens extract with placebo by controlled clinical trial in patients with prostatic adenomatosis. Urologia 50:1257-68, 1983
7. Cirillo-Marucco E, Pagliarulo A, Tritto G, et al: Extract of Serenoa repens (PermixonR) in the early treatment of prostatic hypertrophy. Urologia 5:1269-77, 1983
8. Tripodi V, Giancaspro M, Pascarella M, et al: Treatment of prostatic hypertrophy with Serenoa repens extract. Med Praxis 4:41-6, 1983
9. Emili E, Lo Cigno M and Petrone U: Clinical trial of a new drug for treating hypertrophy of the prostate (Permixon). Urologia 50:1042-8, 1983
10. Greca P and Volpi R: Experience with a new drug in the medical treatment of prostatic adenoma. Urologia 52:532-5, 1985
11. Duvia R, Radice GP and Galdini R: Advances in the phytotherapy of prostatic hypertrophy. Med Praxis 4:143-8, 1983
12. Tasca A, Barulli M, Cavazzana A, et al: Treatment of obstructive symptomatology caused by prostatic adenoma with an extract of Serenoa repens. Double-blind clinical study vs. placebo. Minerva Urol Nefrol 37:87-91, 1985
13. Cukier (Paris), Ducassou (Marseille), Le Guillou (Bordeaux), et al: Permixon versus placebo. C R Ther Pharmacol Clin 4/25:15-21, 1985
14. Champault G, Patel JC and Bonnard AM: A double-blind trial of an extract of the plant Serenoa repens in benign prostatic hyperplasia. Br J Clin Pharmacol 18:461-2, 1984
15. Crimi A and Russo A: Extract of Serenoa repens for the treatment of the functional disturbances of prostate hypertrophy. Med Praxis 4:47-51, 1983
16. Champault G, Bonnard AM, Cauquil J and Patel JC: Medical treatment of prostatic adenoma. Controlled trial: PA 109 vs placebo in 110 patients. Ann Urol 18:407-10, 1984

21

Uva ursi or bearberry

(ARCTOSTAPHYLOS UVA URSI)

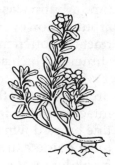

Key uses of uva ursi:
- Urinary tract infections
- Water retention

General description

Uva ursi is a small evergreen shrub found in the northern United States and in Europe. A single long, fibrous main root sends out several prostrate or buried stems 4–6 in. high. The bark is dark brown, the leaves are obovate to spatulate 0.5–1 in. long, the flowers are pink or white and grow in sparse terminal clusters, and the fruit is a bright red or pink.

Chemical composition

Uva ursi's most active ingredient is arbutin, which typically composes 7–9% of the leaves. Other constituents include tannins (6–7%), flavonoids (quercetin), allantoin, gallic and ellagic acids, volatile oils, and the resin urvone.[1,2]

History and folk use

This plant has a long history of use for its diuretic and astringent properties. Conditions for which it was used include urinary tract infections, kidney stones, and bronchitis.[1]

Pharmacology

Pharmacological research has primarily focused on arbutin. In fact, at one time arbutin was marketed as a urinary antiseptic and diuretic. The activity of arbutin, however, is less than that of the total plant.[3] Crude plants or their extracts are often much more effective medicinally than the isolated active constituent, which appears to be the case with uva ursi and arbutin.

For arbutin to be active it must be converted to another compound, hydroquinone, in the urinary tract.[1,2,4] The arbutin molecule must be absorbed intact from the intestine. When arbutin is given alone, bacteria in the intestine break down much of the arbutin before it is absorbed. If the whole plant (or a crude extract) is administered, components in the plant prevent the breakdown of arbutin,[3] which allows for improved absorption of the intact arbutin molecule.[3] The net effect is an increase in the amount of arbutin that is converted to hydroquinone.

The activity of arbutin as an antibiotic in the urinary tract depends on an alkaline urine.[1,2,4] This suggests another reason why the whole plant is of more value than the isolated compound, because the other components of uva ursi make the urine more alkaline.

Dosage

Dosages of three times a day are as follows:

- Dried leaves or by infusion (tea)—1.5–4 g
- Tincture (1:5)—4–6 ml (1–1½ tsp)
- Fluid extract (1:1)—0.5–2.0 ml (⅛–¼ tsp)
- Powdered solid extract (4:1)—250–500 mg

Toxicology

The toxicology of uva ursi is proportional to the conversion of arbutin to hydroquinone. Hydroquinone has been shown to be toxic at 1 g (equivalent to approximately ½ oz of the fresh leaves) with signs and symptoms of tinnitus, nausea, vomiting, sense of suffocation, shortness of breath, cyanosis, convulsions, delirium, and collapse.[2]

References

1. Leung A: Encyclopedia of Common Natural Ingredients Used in Food, Drugs, and Cosmetics. John Wiley & Sons, New York, NY, 1980, pp316-7
2. Merck Index, 10th ed. Merck & Co, Rahway, NJ, 1983 pp796-7 and p4721
3. Frohne V: Untersuchungen zur frage der harndesifizierenden wirkungen von barentraubenblatt-extracten. Planta Medica 18:1-25, 1970
4. Mitchell W: Naturopathic Applications of the Botanical Remedies. Seattle, Wa,1983, p8

SECTION VIII

Herbs for the gastrointestinal tract

The first herb discussed in this section is licorice. Licorice has a broad range of activity and is useful for many other systems of the body. It is included in this section because it has especially significant uses for the gastrointestinal system. Licorice has an impressive ability to heal peptic ulcers.

Chapter 23 highlights the importance of consuming a diet rich in vegetables. As evident in the chapter, fiber possesses tremendously important qualities for maintaining and achieving health, particularly a healthy gastrointestinal tract.

22

Licorice

GLYCYRRHIZA GLABRA

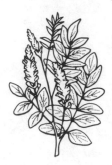

Key uses of licorice:

- Ulcers
- *Herpes simplex* infections
- PMS
- Allergies
- Hepatitis

General description

Glycyrrhiza glabra is a perennial, temperate-zone herb or small shrub, 3–7 ft high, with a long, cylindrical, branched, flexible, and burrowing rootstock with runners. The parts used are the dried runners and roots, which are collected in the fall.

Chemical composition

Licorice root is one of the most extensively investigated botanical medicines. Its major active component is the steroid-like molecule, glycyrrhizin (also known as glycyrrhizic acid or glycyrrhizinic acid), which is found in concentrations of 6–14%. Glycyrrhizin on hydrolysis yields glycyrrhetinic acid and two molecules of glucoronic acid.[1-3]

Other constituents of licorice include flavonoids and isoflavonoids (isoflavonol, kumatakenin, licoricone, glabrol, etc.), chalcones, coumarins (umbelliferone, herniarin, etc.), triterpenoids and sterols, 2–20% starch, 3–14% sugars (glucose, sucrose), lignins, amino acids, amines, gums, and volatile oils.[1-3]

History and folk use

The medicinal use of licorice in both Western and Eastern cultures dates back several thousand years. It was used primarily as a demulcent, an expectorant, an antitussive, and a mild laxative. Licorice is one of the most popular components of Chinese medicines. Its traditional uses include treating peptic ulcers, asthma, pharyngitis, malaria, abdominal pain, insomnia, and infections.[1]

Pharmacology

Licorice is known to exhibit many pharmacological actions, including estrogenic, aldosterone-like action, and anti-inflammatory (cortisol-like) action. It produces antiallergic, antibacterial, antiviral, antitrichomonas, antihepatotoxic, anticonvulsive, choleretic, anticancer, expectorant, and anticough activities.[1-3] Although much of the pharmacology focuses on glycyrrhizin and its aglycone, glycyrrhetinic acid, keep in mind that licorice has many other components, such as flavonoids, which may have significant pharmacological effect.[1-4]

In addition to its medicinal uses, licorice may be used as a pharmaceutical aid. Glycyrrhizin is 50–100 times sweeter than sucrose. Licorice therefore can be used as a sweetening or flavoring agent to mask the bitter taste of other medications.[1,2] The emulsifying activity of its saponins also facilitates the absorption of compounds such as carotenes and anthraquinone glycosides.[2]

Estrogenic activity

Glycyrrhiza exhibits alterative action upon estrogen metabolism (i.e., when estrogen levels are too high, it inhibits estrogen action, and when estrogen levels are too low, it potentiates estrogen action when used in greater amounts.[5] The estrogen action of licorice is a result of its isoflavone content, as well as its glycyrrhetinic acid content. (Many isoflavone structures are known to have an estrogenic effect.)

Pseudoaldosterone activity

Aldosterone is an adrenal hormone responsible for retaining sodium in the body. The chronic ingestion of licorice in large doses leads to a well-documented syndrome which mirrors that of excessive aldosterone, i.e., high blood pressure, high sodium and low potassium levels in the blood, and water retention.[6-8] In normal subjects, the amount of glycyrrhetinic acid needed to produce these side effects is between 0.7 and 1.4 g, which corresponds to approximately 10–14 g of the crude herb.[8] Although licorice possesses aldosterone activity (about four orders of magnitude lower than aldosterone) and binds to aldosterone receptors, it is largely without effect in animals that have had their adrenal glands removed.[9]

G. glabra has been effectively used in the treatment of Addison's disease, a condition of aldosterone insufficiency.[9] Licorice appears to enhance the activity of aldosterone by inhibiting its breakdown by the liver.[10] Glycyrrhizin and glycyrrhetinic acid have been shown to suppress the main enzyme responsible for inactivating cortisol, aldosterone, and progesterone in humans.

Anti-inflammatory and antiallergic activity

Licorice has significant anti-inflammatory and antiallergic activity.[11,12] Although both glycyrrhizin and glycyrrhetinic acid bind to glucocorticoid receptors,[9] and much of licorice's anti-inflammatory activity has been explained by its cortisol-like effects, licorice actually antagonizes the negative effects of cortisol, which stimulates cholesterol synthesis in the liver and damage to the thymus.[13]

The major cortisol-like effect of licorice relates to its ability to inhibit the formation and secretion of inflammatory compounds. In addition, glycyrrhizin has also been shown to inhibit experimentally induced allergenic reactions and to be an antidote against many toxins, including diphtheria, tetanus, and tetrodotoxin.[14,16]

Virtually any inflammatory or allergic condition may be reduced using licorice. Historically, licorice has been used for treating asthma and other atopic conditions.[1,11]

Immunostimulatory and antiviral effects

Glycyrrhizin and glycyrrhetinic acid have been shown to induce interferon production.[17] The induction of interferon leads to significant antiviral activity because interferon binds to cell surfaces, where it stimulates synthesis of intracellular proteins that block viral infection. The induction of interferon is also followed by activation of white blood cells.

Glycyrrhizin has been shown to directly inhibit the growth of several viruses in cell cultures (vaccinia, herpes simplex, Newcastle disease, and vesicular stomatitis viruses) and to inactivate herpes simplex 1 virus irreversibly.[18]

Antibacterial activity

Alcohol extracts of licorice have displayed antimicrobial activity in vitro against *Staphylococcus aureus*, *Streptococcus mutans*, *Mycobacterium smegmatis*, and *Candida albicans*.[19] The majority of the antimicrobial effects are caused by isoflavonoid components, with the saponins having a lesser antibacterial effect.

Licorice in treating peptic ulcer

Besides having a long folk history of use in the treatment of peptic ulcers, glycyrrhitinic acid was the first compound proven to promote the healing of gastric and duodenal ulcers.[21] Its mode of action is different than other medications. Rather than inhibit the release of gastric acid, licorice stimulates the normal defense mechanisms that prevent ulcer formation, which includes increasing the number of mucus-secreting cells (thereby increasing the amount of protective mucosubstances secreted), improving the quality of mucus produced, increasing the life span of the surface intestinal cells, and enhancing the microcirculation of the gastrointestinal tract lining.[23-27,30,39]

Carbenoxolone, a derivative of glycyrrhetinic acid, has been marketed throughout the world for the treatment of both gastric and duodenal ulcers. It has been shown to normalize the disturbance in the structure and function of the intestinal cells caused by cimetidine and has a better effect in preventing ulcer recurrences.[22,28,29] Carbenoxolone and glycyrrhizin have been associated with side effects such as water retention, hypertension, and low potassium levels (pseudoaldosteronism). Because of these known side effects, a procedure was developed to remove glycyrrhizin from licorice to form deglycyrrhizinated licorice (DGL). The result is a very successful antiulcer agent without any known side effects.

Numerous studies over the past 18 years have found DGL to be an effective antiulcer compound. Most of the clinical trials of DGL used a product called Caved-S. This product, available in Europe, has been shown to be very effective in healing peptic ulcers. This form of DGL is supplied in a chewable tablet. It appears that DGL must mix with saliva in order to be effective; another product that contained DGL in capsule form (Ulcedal) was generally ineffective. Ulcedal has been removed from the market.

DGL in treating gastric ulcer

Turpie and colleagues treated 33 gastric ulcer patients with either DGL (760 mg, three times a day) or a placebo for 1 month.[42] There was a significantly greater reduction in ulcer size in the DGL group (78%) than in the placebo group (34%). Complete healing occurred in 44% of those receiving DGL but in only 6% of the placebo group. In another study, DGL promoted healing as effectively as carbenoxolone.[43] DGL was also superior to antacids, with nearly twice as many patients showing complete healing after 6 weeks. This difference, however, was not statistically significant.

DGL has also been shown to be as effective as cimetidine for both short-term treatment and maintenance therapy of gastric ulcer.[44] One hundred patients received either DGL (760 mg, three times a day between meals) or cimetidine (200 mg, three times a day and 400 mg at bedtime). The percentage of ulcers healed after 6 and 12 weeks were similar in both groups. Fifty-six patients received maintenance treatment for 1 year with DGL (760 mg, two times a day) or cimetidine (400 mg at night). The number of recurrences were identical in each group (14%). In another study, DGL was as effective as ranitidine in the treatment of gastric ulcer.[45]

Gastric ulcers are often a result of the use of alcohol, aspirin, or other nonsteroidal anti-inflammatory drugs, or other factors that decrease the integrity of the gastric lining. DGL has been shown to reduce the gastric bleeding caused by aspirin.[46] DGL is strongly indicated for the prevention of gastric ulcers in patients requiring long-term treatment with ulcerogenic drugs, such as aspirin, nonsteroidal anti-inflammatory agents, and corticosteroids.

DGL in treating duodenal ulcer

Forty patients with chronic duodenal ulcers of 4–12 years' duration and more than six relapses during the previous year were treated with DGL.[47] All the patients had been referred for surgery because of relentless pain, sometimes with frequent vomiting, despite treatment with bed rest, antacids, and anticholinergic drugs. Half the patients received 3 g of DGL daily for 8 weeks; the other half received 4.5 g/day for 16 weeks. All 40 patients displayed substantial improvement, usually within 5–7 days, and none required surgery during the 1-year follow-up. Although both dosages were effective, the higher dose was significantly more effective than the lower dose.

In a recent study, the therapeutic effect of DGL was compared to that of antacids, geranylferensylacetate, or cimetidine in 874 patients with endoscopically confirmed chronic duodenal ulceration.[48] Ninety-one percent of all ulcers healed within 12 weeks; there was no significant difference in healing rate among the four groups. However, there were fewer relapses in the DGL group (8.2%) than in those receiving cimetidine (12.9%), geranylferensylacetate (15.5%), or antacids (16.4%). These results, coupled with DGL's protective effects, suggest that DGL may be a more advantageous treatment of duodenal ulcers.

Licorice for treatment of Herpes Simplex

Clinical studies have shown that topical glycyrrhetinic acid and derivatives can be quite helpful in reducing the healing time and pain associated with oral and genital herpes lesions.[31,32] Glycyrrhizin inactivates herpes simplex 1 virus irreversibly and stimulates the synthesis and release of interferon.[17,18]

Acute intermittent porphyria (AIP)

This disorder of heme (the iron-binding protein in blood) biosynthesis is characterized by recurrent attacks of neurological and psychiatric dysfunction.[33,34] The symptoms include abdominal discomfort, nausea, vomiting, and colicky pain, occasionally severe enough to present an acute abdomen without fever or leukocytosis; variable neurological signs and symptoms (e.g., tingling sensations, loss of feeling, neuritic pain, wrist or foot drop, or loss of deep tendon reflexes) and variable mental and emotional disturbances—typically, restlessness, disorientation, and visual hallucinations (experienced by about one-third of the patients). Because estrogens are known to exacerbate or induce AIP, it is quite possible that some of the so-called PMS symptoms are actually a worsening of AIP caused by the mid-cycle estrogen surge. Arsenic and lead can also worsen AIP.[35]

Premenstrual syndrome (PMS)

Besides the association with AIP, PMS symptoms have been largely attributed to an increase in the estrogen:progesterone ratio. Licorice is considered to have alterative action on estrogen metabolism, and both glycyrrhizin and glycyrrhetinic acid have an antiestrogenic effect and may have progesterone-elevating effects also.[5,40] Therefore, licorice may reduce PMS symptoms.

Oral health

Licorice has been a common component in mouthwashes and toothpastes. Although it is 50 to 100 times sweeter than sucrose, glycyrrhizin has significant anticavity effects.[36] Glycyrrhizin has been shown to significantly inhibit plaque growth and bacterial adherence to tooth enamel, in addition to producing antibacterial action against *Streptococcus mutans*, the bacteria largely responsible for cavity development.[36]

Licorice has been reported effective in treating recurrent canker sores. A double-blind cross-over trial demonstrated that a glycyrrhetinic acid mouthwash significantly reduced the average number of mouth ulcers per day, the number of new ulcers that developed, and the discomfort associated with the lesions.[37]

Hepatitis

Glycyrrhizin inhibits liver damage produced by toxic chemicals.[20] Double-blind studies have shown glycyrrhizin effective in treating viral hepatitis, particularly chronic active hepatitis.[14] A glycyrrhizin-containing product (Stronger Neo-minophagen C), consisting of 0.2% glycyrrhizin, 0.1% cysteine, and 2.0% glycine in physiological saline solution, is widely used intravenously in Japan for the treatment of hepatitis.[14] The other components, glycine and cysteine, appear to modulate glycyrrhizin's actions. Glycine has been shown to prevent the aldosterone effects of glycyrrhizin.[14]

Summary

Licorice possesses an impressive spectrum of pharmacological activity, making it useful in a wide range of health conditions. Perhaps its most important therapeutic applications are as an antiulcer medication (in the form of DGL), a tonic useful in treating PMS symptoms and menopausal symptoms, and as an immune-enhancing botanical during viral illness, particularly upper respiratory infections.

Dosages

Dosages of three times a day are as follows:

- Powdered root—1–4 g/day
- Fluid extract (1:1)—4–6 ml (1–1½ tsp)
- Solid (dry powdered) extract (4:1)—250–500 mg
- Deglycyrrhizinated licorice tablets—380–1,140 mg (1–3 chewable tablets)

Toxicology

The main hazard of licorice is its high sodium content and associated water retention. This effect will rarely occur if appropriate precautions are taken. Licorice should not be used by patients who have a history of high blood pressure or renal failure or who currently use heart medicines. There appears to be an individualized response to licorice; therefore blood pressures should be regularly monitored. Prevention of side effects also includes instituting a high-potassium, low-sodium diet. Although no formal trial of either guideline has been performed, patients who normally consume high-potassium foods (fruits and vegetables) and restrict sodium intake—even those patients who have hypertension and angina—have been reported to be free from the aldosterone-like side effects.[38]

References

1. Leung A: Encyclopedia of Common Natural Ingredients Used in Food, Drugs, and Cosmetics. John Wiley & Sons, New York, NY, 1980. pp220-3
2. Tyler V, Brady L and Robbers J: Pharmacognosy, 8th ed. Lea & Febiger, Philadelphia, Pa, 1981. pp68-70
3. Merck Index, 10th ed. Merck & Co, Rahway, NJ 1983. p4374
4. Hattori M, Sakamoto T, Kobashi K, and Namba T: Metabolism of glycyrrhizin by human intestinal flora. Planta Med 48:38-42, 1983
5. Kumagai A, Nishino K, Shimomura A, Kin T, and Yamamura Y: Effect of glycyrrhizin on estrogen action. Endocrinol Japon 14:34-8, 1967
6. Takeda R, Morimoto S, Uchida K, et al: Prolonged pseudoaldosteronism induced by glycyrrhizin. Endocrinol Japon 26:541-7, 1979
7. Baron J: Side-effects of carbonoxolone. Acta Gastro-Enterol Belgica 46:469-84, 1983
8. Epstein M, Espiner E, Donald R, and Hughes H: Effect of eating liquorice on the renin-angiotensin aldosterone axis in normal subjects. Br Med J 1:488-90, 1977
9. Armanini D, Karbowiak I and Funder J: Affinity of liquorice derivatives for mineralocorticoid and glucocorticoid receptors. Clin Endocrinol 19:609-12, 1983
10. Tamura Y, Nishikawa T, Yamada K: Effects of glycyrrhetinic acid and its derivatives on delta4-5-alpha-and 5-beta-reductase in rat liver. Arzneim Forsch 29:647-9, 1979
11. Kuroyanagi T and Sato M: Effect of prednisolone and glycyrrhizin on passive transfer of experimental allergic encephalomyelitis. Allergy 15:67-75, 1966
12. Cyong J: A pharmacological study of the anti-inflammatory activity of chinese herbs. A review. Acupunct Electro-Ther 7:173-202, 1982
13. Kumagai A, Nanaboshi M, Asanuma Y, et al: Effects of glycyrrhizin on thymolytic and immunosuppressive action of cortisone. Endocrinol Japon 14:39-42, 1967
14. Suzuki H, Ohta Y, Takino T, Fujisawa K, et al: Effects of glycyrrhizin on biochemical tests in patients with chronic hepatitis - Double blind trial. Asian Med J 26:423-38, 1984
15. Okimasa E, Moromizato Y, Watanabe S, et al: Inhibition of phospholipase A2 by glycyrrhizin, an anti-inflammatory drug. Acta Med Okayama 37:385-91, 1983
16. Ohuchi K, Kamada Y, Levine L, and Tsurufuji S: Glycyrrhizin inhibits prostaglandin E2 formation by activated peritoneal macrophages from rats. Prostagland Med 7:457-63, 1981
17. Abe N, Ebina T and Ishida N: Interferon induction by glycyrrhizin and glycyrrhetinic acid in mice. Microbial Immunol 26:535-9, 1982
18. Pompei R, Pani A, Flore O, Marcialis M and Loddo B: Antiviral activity of glycyrrhizic acid. Experientia 36:304-5, 1980
19. Mitscher L, Park Y, and Clark D: Antimicrobial agents from higher plants. Antimicrobial isoflavonoids from glycyrrhiza glabra L. var. typica. J Nat Products 43:259-69, 1980
20. Kiso Y, Tohkin M, Hikino H, et al: Mechanism of antihepatotoxic activity of glycyrrhizin, I: effect on free radical generation and lipid peroxidation. Planta Medica 50:298-302, 1984
21. Doll R, Hill I, Hutton C and Underwood D: Clinical trial of a triterpenoid liquorice compound in gastric and duodenal ulcer. Lancet ii:793-6, 1962
22. Capasso F, Mascolo N, Autore G and Duraccio M: Glycyrrhetinic acid, leukocytes and prostaglandins. J Pharm Pharmacol 35:332-5, 1983
23. Symposium international: Peptic ulcer therapy in the 80's. Acta Gastro-Enterol Belgica 46:389-540, 1983
24. Guslandi M: Importance of defensive factors in the prevention of peptic ulcer recurrence. Acta Gastro-Enterol Belgica 46:411-8, 1983
25. Reed P, Vincent-Brown A, Cook P, et al: Comparative study on carbonoxolone and cimetidine in the management of duodenal ulcer. Acta Gastro-Enterol Belgica 46:459-68, 1983
26. Lojda Z and Maratka Z: Histochemistry of the gastroduodenal mucosa under cimetidine and carbonoxolone treatment. Hepatogastroenterol 29:88-9, 1982

27. Moshal M, Gregory M, Pillay C and Spitaels J: Does the duodenal cell ever return to normal? A comparison between treatment with cimetidine and denol. Scand J Gastroenterol 14 (suppl 54):48-51, 1979
28. Boero M, Pera A, Andriulli A, et al: Candida overgrowth in gastric juice of peptic ulcer subjects on short- and long-term treatment with H2-receptor antagonists. Digestion 28:158-163, 1983
29. Johnson B and McIsaac R: Effect of some anti-ulcer agents on mucosal blood flow. Br J Pharmacol i:308, 1981
30. Croft D: Gastric epithelial cell dynamics and the healing of gastric ulcers using carbonoxolone. In: Peptic Ulcer Healing. Recent Studies on Carbonoxolone. Avery Jones F, Langman M and Mann R (eds). MTP Press, Lancaster, UK 1978. pp9-20
31. Partridge M and Poswillo D: Topical carbonoxolone sodium in the management of herpes simplex infection. Br J Oral Maxillofac Surg 22:138-45, 1984
32. Csonka G and Tyrrell D: Treatment of herpes genitalis with carbonoxolone and cicloxolone creams: A double blind placebo controlled trial. Br J Ven Dis 60:178-81, 1984
33. Petersdorf R: Harrison's Principles of Internal Medicine, 10th ed. McGraw-Hill Book Co, New York, NY, 1983. pp535-7
34. Anderson K, Bradlow H, Sassa S, and Kappas A: Studies in porphyria VII. Relationship of the 5-alpha-reductase metabolism of steroid hormones to clinical expression of the genetic defect in acute intermittent porphyria. Am J Med 66:644-50, 1979
35. Tomita T, Sato T, Kazuo S and Takakuwa E: Effects of lead and arsenic on the formation of 5-beta-H steroids. Toxicol Letters 3:291-7, 1979
36. Poswillo D and Partridge M: Management of recurrent aphthous ulcers. Br Dent J 157:55-7, 1984
37. Segal R, Pisanty S, Wormser R, Azaz E and Sela M: Anticarcinogenic activity of licorice and glycyrrhinine I: Inhibition of in vitro plaque formation by streptococcus mutans. J Pharm Sci 74:79-81, 1985
38. Baron J, Nabarro J, Slater J and Tuffley R: Metabolic studies, aldosterone secretion rate and plasma renin after carbonoxolone sodium as biogastrone. Br Med J 2:793-5, 1969
39. Amer S, Mckinney G and Akcasu A: Effect of glycyrrhetinic acid on the cyclic nucleotide system of the rat stomach. Biochem Pharmacol 23:3085-92, 1974
40. Kraus S: The anti-estrogenic action of beta-glycyrrhetinic acid. Exp Med Surg 27:411-20, 1969
41. Sharaf A and Goma N: Phytoestrogens and their antagonism to progesterone and testosterone. J Endocrinol 31:289-90, 1965
42. Turpie AG, Runcie J and Thomson TJ: Clinical trial of deglycyrrhizinate liquorice in gastric ulcer. Gut 10:299-303, 1969
43. Montgomery RD and Cookson JB: The treatment of gastric ulcer. A comparative trial of carbenoxolone and a deglycyrrhizinated liquorice preparation (Caved-S). Clinical Trials Journal 1:33-8, 1972
44. Morgan Ag, McAdam WAF, Pacsoo C and Darnborough A: Comparison between cimetidine and Caved-S in the treatment of gastric ulceration, and subsequent maintenance therapy. Gut 23:545-51, 1982
45. Glick L: Deglycrrhizinated liquorice in peptic ulcer. Lancet ii:817, 1982
46. Rees WDW, Rhodes J, Wright JE, et al: Effect of deglycyrrhizinated liquorice on gastric mucosal damage by aspirin. Scandinavian Journal of Gastroenterology 14:605-7, 1979
47. Tewari SN and Wilson AK: Deglycyrrhizinated liquorice in duodenal ulcer. Practitioner 210:820-5, 1972
48. Kassir ZA: Endoscopic controlled trial of four drug regimens in the treatment of chronic duodenal ulceration. Irish Medical Journal 78:153-6, 1985

23

Dietary fiber

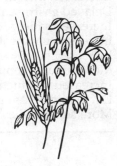

Key uses of fiber:

- Irritable bowel syndrome
- Constipation
- High cholesterol levels
- Obesity

Definition

Currently, the term *dietary fiber* refers to the components of plant cell walls as well as indigestible food residues. The importance of dietary fiber's role in human health is now greatly appreciated (see Table 1).

The composition of the plant cell wall varies according to the species of plant. Typically, the dry cell wall contains 35% cellulose, 45% noncellulose polysaccharides, 17% lignins, 3% protein, and 2% ash.[2,7] It is important to recognize that dietary fiber is a complex of these constituents, and supplementation of a single component does not substitute for a diet rich in high-fiber foods. However, in some clinical conditions the use of specific components is a useful adjunct to a healthy diet. Table 2 summarizes the classifications of dietary fibers.

Cellulose

The best-known component of the plant cell wall is cellulose. Wheat bran is a fiber rich in cellulose. Cellulose is relatively insoluble in water, but it has an ability to bind water, which accounts for its effect of increasing fecal size and weight, thus promoting regular bowel movements. Although cellulose cannot be digested by humans, it is partially digested by the microflora of the

Table 1 Beneficial effects of dietary fiber

Decreased intestinal transit time
Delayed gastric emptying resulting in reduced after-meal elevations of blood sugar
Increased satiety
Increased pancreatic secretion
Increased stool weight
More advantageous intestinal microflora
Increased production of short chain fatty acids
Decreased serum lipids
More soluble bile

digestive tract. This natural fermentation process that occurs in the colon results in the degradation of about 50% of the cellulose and is an important source of short chain fatty acids (SCFA).[2,3] SCFA have very important properties in the colon.

Noncellulose polysaccharides

The majority of polysaccharides in the plant cell wall are of a noncellulose type. They are water-soluble compounds that possess diverse properties (see Table 2). Included in this class are hemicelluloses, gums, mucilages, algal polysaccharides, and pectin substances.[2,3,7]

Hemicelluloses Perhaps the most popular hemicellulose source is oat bran. Hemicelluloses contain a mixture of small sugar molecules (pentose and hexose) in branched-chain configurations of much smaller size than cellulose. The hemicelluloses are more important fiber components than cellulose fibers. They promote regular bowel movements and have many other effects (see Table 2). The hemicelluloses are also a much more important source of SCFA.[2,3,7]

Gums Plant gums are a complex group of water-soluble, gel-forming compounds. They are produced by the plant in response to injury and are commercially produced by incising a plant or tree and collecting the fluid extract. Gums are used as emulsifiers, thickeners, and stabilizers by the food industry and as laxatives in pharmaceuticals.[2,3,7] Examples of plant gums are karaya and gum arabic.

Mucilages Structurally, mucilages resemble the hemicelluloses, but they are not classed as such because of their unique location in the plant. They are

Table 2 Classification of dietary fiber

Fiber class	Chemical structure	Sources	Physiological effects
I. Cellulose	Unbranched 1-4-beta-D glucose polymer	Principle plant wall component Wheat bran	Increases fecal weight and size
II. Noncellulose Polysaccharides			
A. Hemi-cellulose	Mixture of pentose and hexose molecules in branching chains	Plant cell walls Oat bran	Same as above Binds bile acids
B. Gums	Branched chain uronic acid containing polymers	Karaya, gum arabic	Laxative
C. Mucilages	Similar to hemicelluloses	Found in endosperm of plant seeds Guar, legumes, psyllium	Hydrocolloids that bind steroids and delay gastric emptying, heavy metal chelation
D. Pectins	Mixture of methyl-esterified galacturan, galactan, and arabinose in varying proportions	Citrus rind, apple, onion skin	As above
E. Algal Polysaccharides	Polymerized D-mannuronic and L-glucuronic acids	Algin, algin carrageenan	As above
III. Lignans	Noncarbohydrate polymeric phenylpropene	Woody part of plant, wood (40–50%), wheat (25%), apple (25%), cabbage (6%)	Antioxidants, anti-carcinogenic

generally found within the inner layer (endosperm) of the plant seeds, where they are responsible for retaining water to prevent the seed from drying.

Guar gum, found in most beans (legumes), is the most widely studied plant mucilage. Commercially, guar gum is isolated from the endosperm of *Cyamopsis tetragonolobus*, a plant cultivated in India for livestock feed. Guar gum is used commercially as a stabilizer, a thickener, and a film-forming agent in the production of cheese, salad dressings, ice cream, soups, tooth-paste, pharmaceutical jelly, lotion, skin cream, and tablets. Guar gum is also used as a laxative.

Guar gum and other mucilages, including pectin and glucomannan, are perhaps the most potent cholesterol-lowering agents of the gel-forming fibers. Guar gum has been shown to reduce fasting and after-meal glucose and insulin levels in both healthy and diabetic subjects, and it has decreased body weight and hunger ratings when taken with meals by obese subjects.

Psyllium seed husk (plantago ovata) is another mucilage fiber. It is widely used as a bulking and laxative agent and[2,3] possesses many of the same qualities as guar gum, except that it has a greater effect as a laxative.

Algal polysaccharides Included in this fiber category are compounds produced from seaweeds (algae), alginic acid, agar, and carrageenan. These compounds are used extensively by the food industry. Alginate has been shown to inhibit heavy metal uptake in the intestines, as do other gel-forming fibers. Agar is used as a thickening agent and has laxative activity.

Carrageenan is used in milk and chocolate products due to its ability to react with milk proteins. Unlike other plant polysaccharides, carrageenan appears to be detrimental to health.[2,3] In rats, carrageenan has been shown to promote ulceration and damage of the intestines.[3] Other rat studies have shown carrageenan to produce colon cancer, birth defects, and hepato-megaly.[14]

Pectin and pectinlike substances These compounds are found in all plant cell walls as well as in the outer skin and rind of fruits and vegetables. For example, the rind of an orange contains 30% pectin; an apple peel, 15%; and onion skins, 12%.

The gel-forming properties are well known to anyone who has made jelly or jam. These same gel-forming qualities are responsible for the cholesterol-lowering effects of pectins. Pectins lower cholesterol by binding the cholesterol and bile acids in the intestines and promoting their excretion.

Lignans

Lignans are plant products of low molecular weight and typically composed of cinnamic acid, cinnamyl alcohol, propenylbenzene, and allylbenzene precursor units. Many plant lignans show important properties, such as anti-cancer, antibacterial, antifungal, and antiviral activity. Plant lignans are changed by intestinal flora into enterolactone and enterodiol, two compounds believed to protect against cancer, particularly breast cancer.[8]

Miscellaneous fiber-associated compounds

Phytic acid stores minerals such as calcium, phosphorus, magnesium, and potassium in the plant. Dietary phytates adversely affect the uptake and utilization of many minerals, including calcium, iron, and zinc. The major sources of phytate in the diet are cereal grains. However, most of the phytate is destroyed by heat and phytase during the leavening of bread.[2,3,4] Consumption of raw grains or unleavened bread may result in mineral deficiency as a result of the phytates preventing mineral absorption.

Physiological effects of dietary fiber

It is beyond our scope to detail all known effects of dietary fiber on humans. Instead, we will concentrate on the effects of greatest significance (stool weight, transit time, digestion, lipid metabolism, SCFA, and colon flora) and a selection of diseases correlated with the lack of dietary fiber—colon diseases, obesity, and diabetes.

Stool weight and transit time

Fiber has long been used in the treatment of constipation. Dietary fiber, particularly the water-insoluble fibers such as cellulose (e.g., wheat bran), increase stool weight as a result of their water-holding properties.[2-4] Transit time, the time for material to pass from the mouth to the anal canal, is greatly reduced on a high-fiber diet.

Cultures in which the people consume a high-fiber diet (100–170 g/day) usually have a transit time of 30 hr and a fecal weight of 500 g. In contrast, Europeans and Americans who eat a typically low-fiber diet (20 g/day) have a transit time of greater than 48 hr and a fecal weight of only 100 g.[3,7] The increased intestinal transit time associated with the Western diet allows prolonged exposure of various carcinogenic compounds within the intestines.[1-4,12,13]

Fiber should be used not only in the treatment of constipation but also for diarrhea caused by the irritable bowel syndrome. When fiber is added to the diet of subjects who have abnormally rapid transit times (less than 24 hr), the transit time is slowed.[2,3] Dietary fiber acts to normalize bowel movements.

Dietary fiber's effect on transit time is apparently directly related to its effect on stool weight and size. A larger, bulkier stool passes through the colon more easily, requires less pressure to be produced during defecation, and subsequently involves less straining,[1-4] which relieves stress on the colon wall and therefore avoids the ballooning effect, which results in diverticuli. It also prevents the formation of hemorrhoids and varicose veins.

Digestion

Although dietary fiber increases the rate of transit through the gastrointestinal tract, it slows gastric emptying. This results in a more gradual release of food into the small intestine. As a result, blood glucose levels will rise more gradually.[1-4] Pancreatic enzyme secretion and activity also increase in response to fiber.[11]

A number of research studies have examined the effects of fiber on mineral absorption. Although the results have been somewhat contradictory, it now appears that large amounts of dietary fiber may result in impaired absorption and/or negative balance of some minerals. Fiber as a dietary component does not appear to interfere with the minerals in other foods; however, supplemental fiber, especially wheat bran, may result in mineral deficiencies.[2-4]

Lipid metabolism

The water-soluble gels and mucilagenous fibers like oat bran, guar gum, and pectin are capable of lowering serum lipid (i.e., cholesterol and triglyceride) levels by greatly increasing their fecal excretion as well as preventing their manufacture in the liver. The water-insoluble fibers, like wheat bran, have much less effect in reducing serum lipid levels.[1-4]

Short chain fatty acids (SCFA)

The fermentation of dietary fiber by the intestinal flora produces three main end products: (1) short chain fatty acids, (2) various gases, and (3) energy. The SCFAs, acetic, proprionic, and butyric acids, have many important physiological functions. Proprionate and acetate are transported directly to the liver and used for energy production, and butyrate provides an important energy source for the cells that line the colon. In fact, butyrate is the preferred source for energy metabolism in the colon.[2] Butyrate production may also be responsible for the anticancer properties of dietary fiber; it has shown impressive anticancer activity in animals and humans.[2,9,10]

Intestinal bacterial flora

Dietary fiber improves all aspects of colon function.[1-4] Of central importance is the role it plays in maintaining a suitable bacterial flora in the colon. A low-fiber intake is associated with both an overgrowth of endotoxin-producing bacteria ("bad guys") and a lower percentage of lactobacillus ("good guys") and other acid-loving bacteria.[2] A diet high in dietary fiber promotes the growth of acid-loving bacteria through the increased synthesis of SCFA, which reduce the colon pH.

Diseases associated with a lack of dietary fiber

The dietary fiber hypothesis, popularized by the work of Burkitt and Trowell,[1-4] has two basic components: (1) A diet rich in foods that contain plant cell walls (i.e., whole grains, legumes, fruits, and vegetables) protects against a wide variety of diseases, in particular those that are prevalent in Western society; and (2) a diet providing a low intake of plant cell walls is a causative factor in the etiology of these diseases and provides conditions under which other etiological factors are more active.

Although the work of Burkitt and Trowell is well known, it is actually a continuation of the landmark work of Weston A. Price,[5] who brought attention to the "foods of commerce" in the early part of the 20th century. Dr. Price, a dentist, traveled the world observing changes in orthodontic parameters as various cultures discarded traditional dietary practices in favor of a more "civilized" diet. He was able to follow individuals as well as cultures over periods of 20–40 years, and he carefully documented the onset of degenerative diseases as diets changed.

Burkitt formulated the following sequence of events, based on extensive studies examining the rate of diseases in various populations (epidemiological data) and his own observations of primitive cultures:[1,3,4]

> *First stage:* The primal diet of plant eaters contains large amounts of unprocessed starch staples; there are few examples of diseases mentioned in subsequent stages.
>
> *Second stage:* Commencing westernization of diet, obesity and diabetes commonly appear in privileged groups.
>
> *Third stage:* With moderate westernization of the diet, constipation, hemorrhoids, varicose veins, and appendicitis become common clinical entities.
>
> *Fourth stage:* Finally, with full westernization of the diet, ischemic heart disease, diverticular disease, hiatal hernia, and cancer become prominent.

Epidemiological, clinical, and experimental data have linked the Western diet to a number of common diseases. Table 3, prepared from the work of

Table 3 Diseases highly associated with a low-fiber diet

Metabolic	Obesity, gout, diabetes, kidney stones, gallstones
Cardiovascular	Hypertension, cerebrovascular disease, ischemic heart disease, varicose veins, deep vein thrombosis, pulmonary embolism
Colonic	Constipation, appendicitis, diverticulitis, diverticulosis, hemorrhoids, colon cancer, irritable bowel syndrome, ulcerative colitis, Chron's disease
Other	Dental caries, autoimmune disorders, pernicious anemia, multiple sclerosis, thyrotoxicosis, dermatological conditions

Burkitt and Trowell, lists diseases, with convincing documentation, that are linked to a low-fiber diet.[1]

Diseases of the colon

The evidence documenting the protective effect of dietary fiber on colon cancer is overwhelming. There is evidence for similar strong links with other common diseases of the colon—diverticulitis, diverticulosis, irritable bowel syndrome, ulcerative colitis, and appendicitis.[1-4]

Obesity

A diet deficient in dietary fiber is an important causative factor in the development of obesity.[1-4,13] Dietary fiber plays a role in preventing obesity by: (1) increasing the amount of necessary chewing, thus slowing the eating process, (2) increasing fecal caloric loss, (3) improving digestive hormone secretion, (4) improving glucose tolerance, and (5) inducing a state of satiety (feeling of sufficient food intake).

Diabetes mellitus

Population studies and clinical and experimental data show diabetes mellitus to be one of the diseases most clearly related to inadequate dietary fiber intake.[1-4] Clinical studies that have demonstrated the beneficial therapeutic effect of dietary fiber on diabetes have further substantiated this association. Fiber's prevention and improvement of diabetes is due to its effects on glucose and, subsequently, insulin levels.

A high complex-carbohydrate, high-fiber diet reduces after-meal elevations in glucose levels (largely by delaying of gastric emptying and thereby reducing insulin secretion) and increases tissue sensitivity to insulin.[2] Fermentation products of fiber, chiefly SCFA, also enhance liver glucose metabolism and may further contribute to the therapeutic effects of dietary fiber on diabetes.

Summary

A diet high in plant cell walls is associated with a decreased incidence of most of the degenerative diseases of Western society. Although this is largely a result of increased levels of dietary fiber, such a diet is also high in other important nutrients, most of which are also deficient in the Western diet.

It is clear from the scientific literature that the best source of dietary fiber is from whole foods, although specific types of fibers have their use in the treatment phase of specific diseases. Further, even with a diet high in dietary fiber, when as little as 18% of the total calories are in the form of refined carbohydrates, many of the beneficial effects of dietary fiber are greatly reduced.[2] Most Americans consume large amounts of "junk food" loaded with added sugars.[6] There is no substitute for a healthy diet, i.e., a diet composed of foods as close to their original form as possible. However, most people can benefit from supplementing the diet with additional dietary fiber, particularly water-soluble fibers like oat bran and guar gum.

References

1. Burkitt D and Trowell H: Western Diseases: Their Emergence and Prevention. Harvard Univ Press, Cambridge, Mass. 1981
2. Vahouny G and Kritchevsky D: Dietary Fiber in Health and Disease. Plenum Press, New York, NY. 1982
3. Worthington-Roberts B: Contemporary Developments in Nutrition. CV Mosby, St Louis, Mo. 1981
4. Goodhart R and Young VR: Modern Nutrition in Health and Disease. Lea and Febiger, Philadelphia, Pa, 1988
5. Price W: Nutrition and Physical Degeneration. Price-Pottinger Foundation. 1970
6. Linder PG: "Junk foods" and medical education. Obes Bar Med 11:109, 1982
7. Selvendran RR: The plant cell wall as a source of dietary fiber: chemistry and structure. Am J Clin Nutr 39:320-37, 1984
8. Aldercreutz H: Does fiber-rich food containing animal lignan precursors protect against both colon and breast cancer? An extension of the "fiber hypothesis". Gastroen terol 86:761-6, 1984
9. Prasa KN: Butyric acid: A small fatty acid with diverse biological functions. Life Sci 27:1351-8, 1980
10. Novogrodsky A, DVIR A, Ravid A, et al: Effect of polar organic compounds on leukemic cells. Cancer 51:9-14, 1983
11. Sommer H and Kasper H: Effect of long-term administration of dietary fiber on the exocrine pancreas in the rat. Hepato-gastroenterol 31:176-9, 1984
12. National Research Council: Diet, Nutrition and Cancer. National Academy Press. 1982
13. Trowell H: Definition of dietary fiber and hypothesis that it is a protective factor in certain diseases. Am J Clin Nutr 29:417-27, 1976
14. Watt J and Marcus R: Harmful effects of carrageenan fed to animals. Canc Det Prev 4:129-34, 1981

SECTION IX

Herbs for inflammation and arthritis

This section discusses two popular natural anti-inflammatory agents—bromelain and feverfew—which are often used in arthritis and inflammation. They offer an alternative to commonly used anti-inflammatory drugs.

Drugs often are directed against the effects of disease and not the cause. In many instances this suppression of symptoms may actually promote the progression of the disease process. This appears to be the case for the current drug treatment of arthritis—both osteoarthritis and rheumatoid arthritis. In contrast, natural therapy typically is focused against the cause and not simply the effects, or symptoms, of the disease. In the treatment of osteoarthritis, rheumatoid arthritis, and inflammation, there are effective, safe natural approaches.

Osteoarthritis

Osteoarthritis, or degenerative joint disease (DJD) is the most common form of arthritis. It is seen primarily, but not exclusively, in the elderly. Surveys have indicated that over 40 million Americans have osteoarthritis, including

80% of persons over the age of 50. Under the age of 45, osteoarthritis is much more common in men than women. It is 10 times more common in women than men, over the age of 45.

Data collected from the earliest signs of osteoarthritis to the most advanced stages suggest that cellular and tissue response is purposeful and aimed at repair of the damaged joint structure. It appears that the process contributing to osteoarthritis may be arrested and sometimes may be reversed. Therefore, the major therapeutic goal appears to be enhancing repair processes by various joint tissue cells. Nutrition can play a vital role in this process.

Several studies have attempted to determine the "natural course" of osteoarthritis. Perry et al. studied the natural course of osteoarthritis of the hip over a 10-year period.[1] All subjects showed changes suggestive of advanced osteoarthritis, yet the researchers reported marked clinical improvement and radiologic recovery of the joint space in 14 of 31 hips. The authors purposely applied no therapy and regarded their results as reflecting the natural course of the disease.

These results as well as others raise two interesting questions: Does medical intervention in some way promote disease progression? Can various natural therapies enhance the body's own response toward health? The answer to these questions appears to be yes.

The first drug generally used in the treatment of osteoarthritis is aspirin, which is often quite effective in relieving both the pain and the inflammation. It is also relatively inexpensive. However, because the therapeutic dose required is relatively high (2–4 g/day), toxicity often occurs. Tinnitus (ringing in the ears) and gastric irritation (nausea, vomiting, and upset stomach) are early manifestations of toxicity. Chronic use can cause gastric ulcer, kidney damage, liver damage, bleeding disorders, and disturbances to metabolism.

Other nonsteroidal anti-inflammatory drugs (NSAIDs) are often used as well, especially when aspirin is ineffective or intolerable. The following are representative of this class of drugs: ibuprofen (Motrin), fenoprofen (Nalfon), indomethacin (Indocin), naproxen (Naprosyn), tolmetin (Tolectin), and sulindac (Clinoril). These drugs also may cause side effects, including gastrointestinal upset, headaches, and dizziness, and are therefore recommended for only short periods of time.

One side effect of aspirin and other NSAIDs often not mentioned is their inhibition of cartilage repair (i.e., inhibition of collagen matrix synthesis) and acceleration of cartilage destruction. Some experimental studies have revealed this potential side effect.[2] Because osteoarthritis is caused by a degeneration of cartilage, it appears that, although NSAIDs are fairly effective in suppressing the symptoms, they worsen the condition by inhibiting cartilage formation and accelerating cartilage destruction. This has been upheld in studies which have shown that NSAID use is associated with acceleration of osteoarthritis and increased joint destruction.[3-5]

Rheumatoid arthritis

Rheumatoid arthritis (RA) is a chronic inflammatory condition that affects the entire body, including the joints. Between 1 and 3% of the population is affected by RA; female patients outnumber males almost 3:1; and the usual age of onset is 20–40 years, although rheumatoid arthritis may begin at any age.

The first drug generally used in the treatment of RA is also aspirin. As in osteoarthritis, aspirin is often quite effective in relieving both the pain and the inflammation. It also has about the same degree of toxicity. Other NSAIDs may be used as well, especially when aspirin is ineffective or intolerable. None of the other NSAIDs have demonstrated superior efficacy to aspirin, and all are more expensive than aspirin.

There is an interesting association between rheumatoid arthritis and abnormal bowel function. What is currently known is that individuals with RA have increased intestinal permeability to dietary and bacterial antigens as well as alterations in bacterial flora.[6-8] NSAIDs appear to exacerbate the condition. Rheumatoid arthritis is an autoimmune disease in which the body produces antibodies to tissue components (antigens). The permeability and bacterial flora, altered by the ingestion of aspirin or NSAIDs, could result in the absorption of food and microbial antigens that are very similar to antigens in joint tissues. Antibodies formed to bind these antigens would cross-react with the antigens in the joint tissues. Increasingly there is evidence to support this concept.

The natural approach to treating arthritis

Obviously there is a need for a more rational approach to both osteoarthritis and rheumatoid arthritis. A number of natural substances and dietary therapies are more intelligent choices in the treatment of these conditions. The natural approach is more intelligent because it addresses the disease process (i.e, the cause) rather than simply suppressing the symptoms (i.e, the effect).

The natural approach to treating osteoarthritis is to use substances that enhance connective tissue integrity and stimulate repair mechanisms as well as reduce inflammation. Antioxidants, niacin, methionine, trace minerals, flavonoids, and various botanicals, like curcumin and bromelain, are all important in this attempt.

For rheumatoid arthritis, it is necessary to utilize natural measures that reduce the many contributing factors, such as poor digestion, food allergies, increased permeability in the intestines, increased circulating immune complexes, and excessive inflammatory processes. Pancreatic enzymes, hydrochloric acid, EPA (fish oil), selenium, zinc, manganese, bromelain, and various herbal anti-inflammatories like curcumin, bromelain, and feverfew are important considerations in the treatment of RA.

For a more complete discussion of the natural approach to osteo- and rheumatoid arthritis, consult the *Encyclopedia of Natural Medicine*.

References

1. Perry GH, Smith MJG and Whiteside CG: Spontaneous recovery of the hip joint space in degenerative hip disease. Ann Rheum Dis 31:440-8, 1972
2. Brooks PM, Potter SR and Buchanan WW: NSAID and osteoarthritis - help or hindrance. J Rheumatol 9:3-5, 1982
3. Newman, N.M. and Ling, R.S.M. Acetabular bone destruction related to non-steroidal anti-inflammatory drugs. Lancet: ii; 11-13, 1985
4. Solomon L: Drug induced arthropathy and necrosis of the femoral head. J Bone Joint Surg 55B:246-51, 1973
5. Ronningen H and Langeland N: Indomethacin treatment in osteoarthritis of the hip joint. Acta Orthop Scand 50:169-74, 1979
6. Smith MD, Gibson RA and Brooks PM: Abnormal bowel permeability in ankylosing spondylitis and rheumatoid arthritis. Journal of Rheumatology 12:299-305, 1985
7. Zaphiropoulos GC: Rheumatoid arthritis and the gut. British Journal of Rheumatology 25:138-40, 1986
8. Segal AW, Isenberg DA, Hajirousou V, et al: Preliminary evidence for gut involvement in the pathogenesis of rheumatoid arthritis. British Journal of Rheumatology 25:162-6, 1986

24

Bromelain

Key uses of bromelain:

- Inflammation
- Sports injuries
- Respiratory tract infections
- Painful menstruation

General description

Bromelains are sulfur-containing, protein-digesting enzymes (proteolytic enzymes or proteases) obtained from the pineapple plant. Commercial bromelain usually comes from the stem and differs from the bromelain derived from the fruit. Commercial bromelain is a mixture of several proteases and small amounts of several other enzymes and organically bound calcium. Japan, Taiwan, and Hawaii are the major suppliers of commercial bromelain.[1]

History

Bromelain was introduced as a therapeutic agent in 1957. Since that time, over 200 scientific papers on its therapeutic applications have appeared in the medical literature.[2,9] Many of the early studies were performed using Ananase (Rorer), an enteric-coated bromelain tablet. Later studies implied that the failure of bromelain in some of these early studies was a result of the enteric coating as well as inadequate dosages.

Pharmacology

Commercial bromelain has been reported to exert a wide variety of pharmacological effects: assisting digestion, counteracting inflammation, assisting in burn debridement, preventing swelling (edema), relaxing smooth muscle, inhibiting blood platelet aggregation, enhancing antibiotic absorption, preventing ulcers, relieving sinusitis, suppressing appetite, shortening the duration of labor, and enhancing wound healing.[1,2,9] Table 1 highlights conditions for which bromelain may be indicated.

Both stem and fruit bromelains are inhibited by oxidizing agents, such as hydrogen peroxide, methyl bromide, and iodoacetate, and by certain metallic ions, such as lead, mercury, cadmium, copper, and iron. Bromelain protein-digesting activity is also inhibited by human serum. Magnesium and cysteine are activators of commercial bromelain.[1]

The activity of bromelain is expressed in a variety of enzyme units. The use of milk clotting units (m.c.u.) is the officially recognized method in the Food Chemistry Codex (F.C.C.). Different grades of bromelain are available based on m.c.u. For most indications, the recommended m.c.u. range is 1,200–1,800.

Bromelain has been shown to be absorbed via a number of routes and has been effectively administered orally, parenterally, and through intravenous infusion.[3-5] Experiments with dogs have shown oral administration to result in peak levels at 10 hr, but detectable levels are still apparent at 48 hr. Intravenous infusion results in peak levels in 50 min and remains detectable for 5 hr.[4] There is definite evidence that in both animals and people, up to 40% of the absorbed orally administered bromelain can be absorbed intact.[3-5]

Digestive activity

Bromelain is quite effective as a substitute for trypsin or pepsin in cases of pancreatic insufficiency.[2] Because of bromelain's ability to be active in a wide pH range, it can act on substrates in the low pH of the stomach as well as in the high pH of the small intestine. Double-blind studies have shown that the combination of bromelain with pancreatin and ox bile is highly effective in the treatment of pancreatic insufficiency.[6]

Anti-inflammatory activity

Several mechanisms may account for bromelain's anti-inflammatory effects. Hypotheses based on these mechanisms include: (1) activation of proteolytic activity at sites of inflammation (although bromelain's proteolytic actions are inhibited by serum factors), (2) fibrinolysis activity via the plasminogen-

Table 1 Conditions in which bromelain has documented clinical efficacy[1-34]

Angina	Maldigestion
Arthritis	Pancreatic insufficiency
Athletic injury	Phytobezoar
Bronchitis	Pneumonia
Burn debridement	Scleroderma
Cellulitis	Sinusitis
Dysmenorrhea	Staphylococcal infection
Ecchymosis	Surgical trauma
Edema	Thrombophlebitis

plasmin system, (3) depletion of kininogen, and (4) inhibition of biosynthesis of proinflammatory prostaglandins and induction of prostaglandin E_1 accumulation (which tends to inhibit the release of PMN lysosomal enzymes).[7-9]

The first hypothesis has not been substantiated; the remaining three hypotheses may be part of the same mechanism of action. After tissue injury, the kinin, complement, fibrinolytic, and clotting systems are activated. These systems are closely interrelated via activation of the Hageman factor (XII) and feedback mechanisms.

Fibrin's role in promoting the inflammatory response is to form a matrix that walls off the area of inflammation, resulting in blockage of blood vessels, inadequate tissue drainage, and edema; the kinin system cascade causes the production of kinins (e.g., bradykinin and kallidin). These compounds increase vascular permeability, causing edema and pain.

Bromelain's first effect in reducing inflammation is to break down fibrin, a process known as fibrinolysis. Bromelain does this by stimulating plasmin production, which breaks down the fibrin, thereby eliminating fibrin's effect of preventing tissue drainage and producing localized swelling.[7,8,32,33] Plasmin has been shown to block the formation of proinflammatory compounds.[12]

Bromelain has also been shown to reduce plasma kininogen levels. The net result of this action is inhibition of the production of kinins.[10] Because kinins cause much inflammation, swelling, and pain, inhibiting their production is warranted in traumatic injuries like sports injuries.

These actions—the activation of plasmin and the reduction of kinin levels—are probably the main pharmacological effects of bromelain. Bromelain's ability to reduce inflammation has been documented in a variety of experimental models and clinical studies.

Antibiotic activity

Clinical studies have shown that bromelain increases serum levels of a variety of antibiotics (e.g., amoxycillin, tetracycline, and penicillin) in many different tissues and body fluids (e.g., cerebral spinal fluid, sputum, mucus, blood, urine, uterus, salpinx, ovary, gallbladder, appendix, and epithelial tissue).[22-24] In these studies, the researchers concluded that bromelain itself possesses significant effects. Bromelain is as effective as antibiotics in treating a variety of infectious processes, i.e., pneumonia, perirectal abscess, cutaneous staphylococcal infection, pyelonephritis, and bronchitis.[22]

Bromelain in respiratory tract diseases

In the treatment of chronic bronchitis, bromelain was shown to have an antitussive effect (suppression of cough) and to reduce the viscosity of sputum. Examination of patients using a specialized apparatus for determining respiratory function (a spirometer) before and after treatment indicated increased lung capacity and function. These favorable effects were believed to be the results of enhanced resolution of respiratory congestion, due to bromelain's ability to fluidify and decrease bronchial secretions. It appears that bromelain's mucolytic activity is responsible for its particular effectiveness in treating respiratory tract diseases.[25] Acute sinusitis has also responded to bromelain therapy. Good to excellent results were obtained in 87% of bromelain-treated patients, compared with 68% of the placebo group.[26]

Thrombophlebitis

Numerous investigators have demonstrated that orally administered bromelain has a very favorable effect on acute thrombophlebitis (inflammation of a vein), deep vein thrombosis, cellulitis, bruises, and edema.[13-16] In a double-blind study involving 73 patients with acute thrombophlebitis, bromelain, as an adjunct to analgesics, was shown to reduce all the symptoms of inflammation: pain, edema, redness, tenderness, elevated skin temperature, and disability.[14] In this study and others, the common daily dose of bromelain was 60–160 mg of 1,200 m.c.u. bromelain. According to some researchers, doses of 400–800 mg are needed to achieve consistent results in patients with thrombophlebitis; this probably holds true for most other conditions.[13]

Surgical procedures and athletic injuries

The effect of orally administered bromelain on the reduction of swelling, bruising, healing time, and pain following various surgical procedures has been demonstrated in several clinical studies.[17-20] Tassman's studies of patients undergoing oral surgery concluded that although after-surgery medication alone is effective, a regimen of before-and-after surgery medication is recommended.[17,18]

In one double-blind study of patients undergoing oral surgery, bromelain was found to be significantly superior to placebo: swelling decreased in 3.8 days with bromelain, compared with 7 days for the placebo; and the duration of pain was reduced to 5.1 days in the bromelain group, compared with 8.1 in the placebo.[18] Similar observations were made in studies of episiotomy cases. Bromelain reduced edema, inflammation, and pain, and preoperative administration potentiated the effects.[19,20]

Bromelain has been used in a variety of sports-related injuries. A 1960 study involving boxers highlights the effects of bromelain.[21] Among the 74 boxers receiving bromelain, all signs of bruising cleared completely within 4 days for 58 boxers. For the remainder, complete clearance took 8–10 days. Among the 72 controls, at the end of 4 days only 10 showed bruises completely cleared, the remainder taking 7–14 days. It is important to recognize that although bromelain has been shown to effectively reduce pain, this probably is the result of a reduction in tissue inflammation and edema rather than a direct analgesic effect.

Dysmenorrhea

Bromelain and papain have been used successfully in the treatment of dysmenorrhea (painful menstruation).[27] Bromelain is believed to be a smooth muscle relaxant because it decreases the spasms of the contracted cervix in these patients. Failure of the bromelain protease to produce this effect was the first indication that the pharmacologically important factor may not be the main protease.

Summary

Bromelain has a wide range of therapeutic utility. It is effective in virtually all inflammatory conditions, regardless of cause, including those resulting from physical trauma, infectious agents, surgical procedures, and autoimmune mechanisms.

Dosage

Unless bromelain is being used as a digestive aid, it should be taken on an empty stomach (between meals). The dosage depends largely on the potency of the bromelain preparation. Most currently available bromelain is in the 1,200–1,800 m.c.u. range. The typical dosage is 250–500 mg three times a day.

Toxicology

Very large doses of bromelain (nearly 2.0 g) have been given with no side effects.[28] It is virtually nontoxic because no LD_{50} exists up to 10 g/kg. Chronic use appears to be well tolerated. Although no significant side effects have been noted, as with most therapeutic agents, allergic reactions may occur in sensitive individuals or with prolonged occupational exposure.[29,30] Other possible but unconfirmed reactions include nausea, vomiting, diarrhea, metrorrhagia, and menorrhagia.[31]

References

1. Leung A: Encyclopedia of Common Natural Ingredients Used in Foods, Drugs, and Cosmetics. John Wiley & Sons, New York, NY, 1980. pp74-6
2. Taussig S, Yokoyama M, Chinen A, et al: Bromelain, a proteolytic enzyme and its clinical application. A review. Hiroshima J Med Sci 24:185-93, 1975
3. Miller J and Opher A: The increased proteolytic activity of human blood serum after oral administration of bromelain. Exp Med Surg 22:277-80, 1964
4. Izaka K, Yamada M, Kawano T and Suyama T: Gastrointestinal absorption and anti-inflammatory effect of bromelain. Jap J Pharmacol 22:519-34, 1972
5. Seifert J, Ganser R and Brendel W: Absorption of a proteolytic enzyme of plant origin from the gastrointestinal tract into the blood and lymph of adult rats. Z Gastroenterol 17:1-18, 1979
6. Balakrishnan V, Hareendran A and Nair C: Double-blind cross-over trial of an enzyme preparation in pancreatic steatorrhoea. J Assoc Phys Ind 29:207-9, 1981
7. Ako H, Cheung A and Matsura P: Isolation of a fibrinolysis enzyme activator from commercial bromelain. Arch Int Pharmacodyn. 254:157-167, 1981
8. Taussig S: The mechanism of the physiological action of bromelain. Med Hypothesis 6:99-104, 1980
9. Felton G: Does kinin released by pineapple stem bromelain stimulate production of prostaglandin E1-like compounds? Hawaii Med J 36:39-47, 1977
10. Katori M, Ikeda K, Harada Y, et al: A possible role of prostaglandins and bradykinin as a trigger of exudation in carrageenin-induced rat pleurisy. Agents Actions 8:108-12, 1978
11. Heinicke R, van der Wal L and Yokoyama M: Effect of bromelain (Ananase) on human platelet aggregation. Experentia 28:844-5, 1972
12. Schafer A and Adelman B: Plasmin inhibition of platelet function and of arachidonic acid metabolism. J Clin Invest 75:456-461, 1985
13. Taussig S and Nieper H: Bromelain: Its use in prevention and treatment of cardiovascular disease present status. J Int Assoc Prev Med 6:139-51, 1979
14. Seligman B: Oral bromelains as adjuncts in the treatment of acute thrombophlebitis. Angiology 20:22-6, 1969
15. Seligman B: Bromelain: An anti-inflammatory agent. Angiology 13:508-10, 1962
16. Felton G: Fibrinolytic and antithrombotic action of bromelain may eliminate thrombosis in heart patients. Med Hypothesis 6:1123-33, 1980
17. Tassman G, Zafran J and Zayon G: Evaluation of a plant proteolytic enzyme for the control of inflammation and pain. J Dent Med 19:73-7, 1964
18. Tassman G, Zafran J and Zayon G: A double-blind crossover study of a plant proteolytic enzyme in oral surgery. J Dent Med 20:51-4, 1965

19. Howat R and Lewis G: The effect of bromelain therapy on episiotomy wounds - A double blind controlled clinical trial. J Ob Gyn Brit Commonwealth 79:951-3, 1972
20. Zatuchni G and Colombi D: Bromelains therapy for the prevention of episiotomy pain. Ob Gyn 29:275-8, 1967
21. Blonstein J: Control of swelling in boxing injuries. Practitioner 203:206, 1960
22. Neubauer R: A plant protease for the potentiation of and possible replacement of antibiotics. Exp Med Surg 19:143-60, 1961
23. Luerti M and Vignali M: Influence of bromelain on penetration of antibiotics in uterus, salpinx and ovary. Drugs Exp Clin Res 4:45-8, 1978
24. Tinozzi S and Venegoni A: Effect of bromelain on serum and tissue levels of amoxycillin. Drugs Exp Clin Res 4:39-44, 1978
25. Rimoldi R, Ginesu F and Giura R: The use of bromelain in pneumological therapy. Drugs Exp Clin Res 4:55-66, 1978
26. Ryan R: A double-blind clinical evaluation of bromelains in the treatment of acute sinusitis. Headache 7:13-7, 1967
27. Hunter RG, Henry GW and Henicke RM: The action of papain and bromelain on the uterus. Am J Ob Gyn 73:867-880, 1957
28. Gutfreund A, Taussig S and Morris A: Effect of oral bromelain on blood pressure and heart rate of hypertensive patients. Hawaii Med J 37:143-6, 1978
29. Baur X: Studies on the specificity of human IgE-antibodies to the plant proteases papain and bromelain. Clinical Allergy 9:451-7, 1979
30. Baur X and Fruhman G: Allergic reactions, including asthma, to the pineapple protease bromelain following occupational exposure. Clinical Allergy 9:443-50, 1979
31. Physicians Desk Reference: Ananase (Rorer). Medical Economics Company, 1982. p1645
32. Pirotta F and de Giuli-Morghen C: Bromelain - A deeper pharmacological study. Note I - Anti-inflammatory and serum fibrinolytic activity after oral administration in the rat. Drugs Exp Clin Res 4:1-20, 1978
33. de Giuli-Morghen C and Pirotta F: Bromelain - A deeper pharmacological study. Note II - Interaction with some protease inhibitors and rabbit specific antiserum. Drugs Exp Clin Res 4:21-37, 1978
34. Ballard T: Bromelain. J John Bastyr Col Nat Med 1:37-41, 1979

25

Feverfew
(TANACETUM PARTHENIUM)

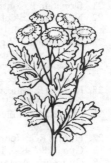

Key uses of feverfew:

- Migraine headaches
- Arthritis
- Fever
- Inflammation

General description

Feverfew (a corruption of the word *febrifuge*, from its tonic and fever-dispelling properties) is a composite plant that is cultivated throughout Europe and the United States. The round, leafy, branching stems bear alternate, bipinnate leaves with ovate, hoary-green leaflets. The flowers are small and daisylike, with yellow disks and 10–20 white, toothed rays.

Chemical composition

The plant is rich in sesquiterpene lactones, principally parthenolide. The flowering herb also contains 0.02–0.07% essential oils (L-camphor, L-borneol, terpenes, and miscellaneous esters).[1,2]

History and folk use

Feverfew has been used for centuries as a febrifuge and for the treatment of migraines and arthritis. Other historical uses of feverfew have been in the treatment of anemia, earache, dysmenorrhea, dyspepsia, trauma, and intestinal parasites.[1] Feverfew has been used to induce abortion. In addition, it has been used in gardens to control noxious pests. (Its pyrethrin component is an effective insecticide.)[7]

Pharmacology

Anti-inflammatory effects

Feverfew has demonstrated some remarkable pharmacological effects in experimental studies. Its long folk history of use in the treatment of inflammatory conditions such as fever, arthritis, and migraine suggests that it acts in a fashion similar to that of the more common NSAIDs, such as aspirin, which reduce the production of inflammatory compounds. Extracts of feverfew have actually been shown to inhibit the synthesis of these inflammatory compounds to a much greater degree than aspirin.

Feverfew also produces an effect that aspirin does not—an ability to reduce the secretion of inflammatory particles by platelets and white blood cells. This is particularly important in the treatment of rheumatoid arthitis, a condition characterized by tremendous inflammation, largely the result of platelets and white blood cells releasing inflammatory particles; and the treatment of migraine headache, a condition linked to the release of serotonin by blood platelets. Serotonin released by platelets causes spasms of the blood vessel and migraine headache.

Platelet aggregation inhibition

Currently, many physicians are recommending daily aspirin use as a preventive measure against strokes and heart attacks because aspirin is able to inhibit platelets from aggregating and forming clots. Presumably, feverfew could also be used in this manner. This herb has demonstrated remarkable effects on platelets.[3-5]

Feverfew in migraine headaches

In a recent survey it was discovered that 70% of 270 migraine sufferers who had eaten feverfew daily for prolonged periods claimed that the herb decreased the frequency or intensity of their migraine attacks.[6] Many of these patients had been unresponsive to orthodox medications.

The therapeutic and preventive effect of feverfew in the treatment of migraine headache displayed in this survey led to a controlled double-blind study at the London Migraine Clinic, using patients who reported to be helped by feverfew.[6] The results of this 6-month double-blind study were very encouraging. Those patients who received the placebo had a significant increase in the frequency and severity of headache, nausea, and vomiting during the 6 months of the study. Patients who took feverfew showed no change in the frequency or severity of their symptoms. Two patients in the placebo group who had been in complete remission during self-treatment with feverfew leaves developed recurrence of incapacitating migraine and had to withdraw from the study. Resuming self-treatment with feverfew resulted in the remission of migraine in both patients.

Feverfew in rheumatoid arthritis

Inflammatory compounds released by white blood cells and platelets contribute greatly to the inflammation and cellular damage found in rheumatoid arthritis. The inhibition of the release of inflammatory particles by feverfew is much greater than that achieved by NSAIDs like aspirin.[5] This factor, coupled with many of feverfew's other effects, indicate that feverfew could greatly reduce inflammation in rheumatoid arthritis.

A double-blind, placebo-controlled study demonstrated no apparent benefit from orally administered feverfew in RA patients. However, the dosage used was extremely small (76 mg dried, powdered feverfew leaf corresponding to two medium-sized leaves). In addition, patients had continued to take NSAIDs during the study—a practice that has been suggested to reduce the efficacy of feverfew.[9]

Future applications of feverfew

Further clinical studies on feverfew are expected in the near future. From the experimental data, feverfew appears to be indicated in conditions that are typically treated with NSAIDs. Included in this category is the use of feverfew as a febrifuge or antipyretic. The doctrine of signatures appears to be upheld in the case of feverfew because its root is reported to taste hot.[8]

Summary

Feverfew possesses significant anti-inflammatory action and may provide substantial relief in cases of migraine and rheumatoid arthritis.

Dosage

The dosage used in the migraine study was 25 mg of the dried leaves twice a day, which appeared adequate in the prevention of migraines. The standard three-times a day dosages are as follows:

- Dried leaves or by infusion (tea)—1–2 g
- Tincture (1:5)—4–6 ml (1–1½ tsp)
- Fluid extract (1:1)—1–2.0 ml (¼–½ tsp)
- Powdered solid extract (4:1)—250–500 mg

Toxicology

There were no reports of toxic reactions in patients taking feverfew in the 6-month migraine study. Feverfew has been used by large numbers of people for many years without reports of toxicity. Chewing the leaves, however, may result in canker sores, and some sensitive persons will develop a rash if feverfew touches their skin [7]

References

1. Duke JA: Handbook of Medicinal Herbs. CRC Press, Boca Raton, Fl 1985. p118
2. Bohlmann F and Zdero C: Sesquiterpene lactones and other constituents from Tanacetum parthenium. Phytochemistry 21:2543-9, 1982
3. Makheja AM and Bailey JM: The active principle in feverfew. Lancet ii:1054, 1981
4. Makheja AM and Bailey JM: A platelet phospholipase inhibitor from the medicinal herb feverfew (Tanacetum parthenium). Prostagland Leukotri Med 8:653-60, 1982
5. Heptinstall S, White A, Williamson L and Mitchell JRA: Extracts of feverfew inhibit granule secretion in blood platelets and polymorphonuclear leukocytes. Lancet i:1071-4, 1985
6. Johnson ES, Kadam NP, Hylands DM, and Hylands PJ: Efficacy of feverfew as prophylactic treatment of migraine. Br Med J 291:569-73, 1985
7. Dreisbach RH: Handbook of Poisoning, 11th ed. Lange Med Publ, Los Altos, Ca, 1983. p552
8. Lewis WH and Elvin-Lewis MPF: Medical Botany. John Wiley & Sons, New York, NY, 1977. p323,368
9. Pattrick M, Heptinstall S and Doherty M: Feverfew in rheumatoid arthritis: A double blind, placebo controlled study. Annals Rheum Dis 48:547-9, 1989

SECTION X

Herbal sedatives

This section describes valerian and St John's wort, two popular herbs used in the treatment of insomnia. Within the course of a year, up to 30% of the population suffers from insomnia. Many people use over-the-counter medications to combat the problem, whereas others seek stronger sedatives. Each year, 4 million to 6 million people in the United States receive prescriptions for sedative hypnotics.

Various compounds in food and drink can interfere with normal sleep, including stimulants, thyroid preparations, oral contraceptives, beta-blockers, marijuana, alcohol, coffee, tea, and chocolate. Insomnia is a symptom that can have many causes. The following chart lists some of the more common causes of insomnia.

CAUSES OF INSOMNIA

Anxiety or tension	Sleep apnea
Environmental change	Nocturnal myoclonus
Emotional arousal	Hypoglycemia
Fear of insomnia	Parasomnias
Phobia of sleep	Caffeine
Disruptive environment	Drugs
Pain or discomfort	Alcohol
Depression	

The naturopathic approach to insomnia is to address the cause before simply prescribing a natural sedative. When indicated, natural sedatives like valerian and St. John's wort are actually more effective than over-the-counter or prescription sedatives. The problem with the synthetic sedatives is that they tend to interfere with normal sleep processes. The result is that the individual may feel more exhausted on waking up in the morning than when he or she went to bed. In contrast, herbal sedatives appear to enhance sleep processes without producing a "hangover" effect.

26

Valerian

(VALERIANA OFFICINALIS)

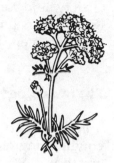

Key uses of valerian:

- Insomnia
- Anxiety
- High blood pressure
- Intestinal spasm

General description

Valerian is a perennial plant native to North America and Europe. The yellow-brown tuberous rootstock produces a flowering stem 2–4 ft high. The stem is grooved, and hollow; leaves are arranged in pairs. The small rose-colored flowers are in bloom from June to September. The rootstock is the portion used medicinally.

Chemical composition

The important active compounds of valerian are the so-called valepotriates (iridoid molecules) and valeric acid, found exclusively in valerian. Originally, it was thought that just the valepotriates were responsible for valerian's sedative effects, but recently an aqueous extract of valerian was shown to have sedative effects. Because the valepotriates are not water-soluble, researchers concluded that valeric acid also possesses sedative action. Valeric acid is believed to be the chemical factor responsible for the sedative effect noted in human clinical trials that used an aqueous extract of valerian root. Other components of valerian include a volatile oil (0.5–2%), choline (3%), flavonoids, sterols, and various alkaloids.[1]

History and folk use

Historically, valerian's prime use was as a sedative in the relief of insomnia, anxiety, and conditions associated with pain. Specific conditions for which it was used include migraine, insomnia, hysteria, fatigue, intestinal cramps, and other nervous conditions.

Pharmacology

Valerian has demonstrated a number of pharmacological effects. It has an equilibrating effect on the central nervous system, as a sedative in states of agitation and as a stimulant in cases of extreme fatigue. This herb also demonstrates blood pressure lowering effects, an ability to enhance the flow of bile (choleretic effect), the ability to relax intestinal muscle, and antitumor and antibiotic activity.[2-5] Its prime pharmacological effect, however, is consistent with its historical use, i.e., as a sedative.

Recent scientific studies have substantiated valerian's ability to improve sleep quality and relieve insomnia.[6,7] A double-blind study involving 128 subjects showed that an aqueous extract of valerian root improved the subjective ratings for sleep quality and sleep latency (the time required to get to sleep) but left no "hangover" effect in the next morning.[6]

In a follow-up study, valerian extract was shown to significantly reduce sleep latency, improve sleep quality, and reduce nighttime awakenings in sufferers of insomnia. This study was performed under strict laboratory conditions. The results of the study indicate that valerian is as effective in reducing sleep latency as small doses of barbiturate or benzodiazepans.[7] The difference, however, is that these chemical compounds increase morning sleepiness. Valerian, on the other hand, actually reduces morning sleepiness. The results were confirmed in a subsequent double-blind placebo-controlled study.[8]

Summary

Valerian is a safe and effective sleep-promoting aid.

Dosage

As a mild sedative, valerian may be taken at the following dose, 30–45 min before retiring:

- Dried root (or as tea)—1–2 g
- Tincture (1:5)—4–6 ml (1–1.5 tsp)
- Fluid extract (1:1)—1–2 ml (0.5–1 tsp)
- Solid (dried powdered) extract (4:1)—250–500 mg
- Valerian extract (1.0–1.5% valtrate or 0.8% valeric acid)—150–300 mg

If morning sleepiness results, a reduction in dosage is recommended. If dosage is not effective, the user should make sure he or she has eliminated those factors that disrupt sleep, such as caffeine and alcohol.

Toxicology

Valerian is generally regarded as safe and is approved for food use by the U.S. Food and Drug Administration.[1]

References

1. Leung A: Encyclopedia of Common Natural Ingredients Used in Food, Drugs, and Cosmetics. John Wiley & Sons, New York, NY
2. Takeda S, Endo T and Aburada M: Pharmacological studies on iridoid compounds. III. The choleretic mechanism of iridoid compounds. J Pharm Dyn 4:612-23, 1981
3. Hendriks H, Bos R, Allersma DP, et al: Pharmacological screening of valerenal and some other components of essential oil of valeriana officinalis. Planta Medica 42:62-8, 1981
4. Hazelhoff B, Malingre TM and Meijer DK: Antispamodic effects of valeriana compounds: an in-vivo and in vitro study on the guinea pig ileum. Arch Int Pharmacodyn 257:274-87, 1982
5. Bounthanh C, Bergmann C, Beck JP, et al: Valepotriates, a new class of cytotoxic and antitumor agents. Planta Medica 41:21-8, 1981
6. Leathwood P, Chauffard F, Heck E, and Munoz-Box R: Aqueous extract of valerian root (Valeriana officinalis L.) improves sleep quality in man. Pharmacol Biochem Behavior 17:65-71, 1982
7. Leathwood PD and Chauffard F: Aqueous extract of valerian reduces latency to fall asleep in man. Planta Medica 54:144-8, 1985
8. Lindahl O and Lindwall L: Double blind study of a valerian preparation. Pharmacol Biochem Behavior 32:1065-6, 1989

27

St. John's wort

(HYPERICUM PERFORATUM)

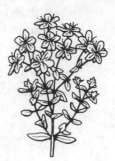

Key uses of St. John's wort:

- Depression
- Anxiety
- Sleep disturbance
- Aids

General description

St. John's wort, or *Hypericum*, is a shrubby perennial plant commonly found in dry, gravelly soils, in fields and other sunny places. St. John's wort is native to many parts of the world, including Europe and the United States. It grows especially well in northern California and southern Oregon.

Chemical composition

The leaves and flowers of *Hypericum* contain a complex and diverse mixture of chemical compounds. The dianthrone derivatives, hypericin and pseudo-hypericin, are of great interest for their pharmacological activity. Other active components include flavonoids, xanthones, phenolic carboxylic acids, essential oils, carotenoids, alkanes, and phloroglucinol derivatives.

History and folk use

Hypericum has a long history of use. Dioscorides, the foremost physician of ancient Greece, as well as Pliny and Hippocrates, used this plant to treat many illnesses. Its botanical name, *Hypericum perforatum,* is derived from its Greek name, which means "over an apparition"; the herb was believed to be so obnoxious to evil spirits that a whiff of it would cause them to fly.

The plant's common name has been attributed to several events or beliefs. Some myths claim that red spots, symbolic of the blood of St. John, appeared on the leaves of a *Hypericum* plant on the anniversary of the saint's beheading. There was also a common medieval belief that if one slept with a piece of the plant under one's pillow on St. John's Eve, the Saint would appear in a dream, give his blessing, and prevent one from dying during the following year.

Many people, from the time of the ancient Greeks through the Middle Ages, believed that St. John's wort has magical powers. Recent research is discovering why. From this research, it appears that St. John's wort will continue to be a highly respected herb for many more years to come.

In Europe, St. John's wort has a long history of use, particularly as a folk remedy in the treatment of wounds, kidney and lung ailments, and depression.[1]

Pharmacology

Mood-elevating effects

One of the most popular historical uses of St. John's wort was as a mood elevator, in cases of depression and other mental illness. Researchers have discovered that components in St. John' wort do, in fact, alter brain chemistry in a way which improves mood.[2] A clinical study of 15 women with depression demonstrated that a standardized extract of St. John's wort led to significant improvement in symptoms of anxiety, depression, and feelings of worthlessness.[3] In addition, the extract greatly improved sleep quality because it was effective in relieving both insomnia and hypersomnia (excessive sleep).

Antiviral effects

A tremendous amount of excitement about St. John's wort occurred after researchers from New York University Medical Center and the Weizmann Institute of Science in Israel demonstrated in a preliminary study that the St. John's wort components, hypericin and pseudohypericin, inhibit a variety of retroviruses, including the retrovirus associated with AIDS (the human immunodeficiency virus, or HIV).

The researchers concluded:

Hypericin and pseudohypericin display an extremely effective antiviral activity when administered to mice after retroviral infection. . . . The antiviral activity is remarkable both in its mechanism of action . . . and in the potency of one administration of a relatively small dose of the compounds. Availability . . . and the relatively convenient and inexpensive procedure for the extraction and purification of hypericin and pseudohypericin further enhance the potential of these compounds.[4]

Many questions must be answered before St. John's wort can be recommended as a supportive measure in the treatment of AIDS, but this information certainly is encouraging.

Summary

St. John's wort has been a highly respected plant medicine for thousands of years. In earlier times, its effects were thought to be magical. However, modern research is providing an explanation for many of these magical effects.

Research suggests a possible role in the treatment of AIDS because of its retrovirus-inhibiting activity. At this time, however, St. John's wort cannot be recommended for treating AIDS. The primary use of St. John's wort or its extracts at this time is in psychological complaints such as mild depression, anxiety, and sleep disturbances.

Dosage

Dosages of three times a day are as follows:

- Dried herb as infusion (tea)—1–2 g
- Tincture (1:5)—3–6 ml (¾–1½ tsp)
- Fluid extract (1:1)—0.5–1 ml (⅛–¼ tsp)
- Solid (powdered dry) extract (5:1 or 0.125% hypericin)—125–250 mg

Toxicology

Although there is considerable evidence that St. John's wort can cause severe photosensitivity in animals grazing extensively on the plant, there is no evidence that St. John's wort is toxic to humans, especially when used at recommended medicinal doses. Nonetheless, some herbalists recommend that individuals avoid exposure to strong sunlight when using St. John's wort.[1]

References

1. Hobbs C: St. John's Wort, Hypericum perforatum L. HerbalGram 18/19:24-33, 1989
2. Suzuki O, et al.:Inhibition of monoamine oxidase by hypericin. Planta Medica 50:272-4, 1984
3. Muldner VH and Zoller M: Antidepressive wirkung eines auf den wirkstoffkomplex hypericin standardisierten hypericum-extrakes. Arzneim Forsch 34:918, 1984
4. Meruelo D, et al.: Therapeutic agents with dramatic antiretroviral activity and little toxicity at effective doses: Aromatic polycyclic diones hypericin and pseudohypericin. Proceedings National Academy of Sciences 85:5230-34, 1988

SECTION XI

Herbs for the skin

Herbal compounds have long been used in cosmetics and skin products. Rather than highlight the many cosmetic effects of herbs, this section highlights the medical use of three herbs commonly used in skin complaints: gotu kola, sarsaparilla, and tea tree oil. All three herbs in this section have an interesting history and folk use.

Gotu kola is a particularly interesting herb for the skin because it increases the blood supply to the dermis, which is the support structure of the skin. Many minor skin complaints will disappear as a result of using this herb. Many women are fond of gotu kola because of its ability to improve the appearance of cellulite.

28

Gotu kola

(CENTELLA ASIATICA)

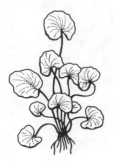

Key uses of gotu kola:

- Cellulite
- Wound healing
- Varicose veins
- Scleroderma

General description

Centella asiatica, or gotu kola, is a perennial plant native to India, China, Indonesia, Australia, the South Pacific, Madagascar, and southern and middle Africa. It is a slender, creeping plant that flourishes in and around water. Although it grows best in damp, swampy areas, gotu kola often grows along stone walls or other rocky, sunny areas at elevations of approximately 2,000 ft in India and Ceylon.[1]

Depending on environmental circumstances, the form and shape of *Centella* changes dramatically. In shallow water, the plant will form with only floating leaves, whereas in dry locations numerous roots are formed and the leaves are small and thin.[1]

Typically, the constantly growing roots give rise to reddish, string-shaped stolons. The round to kidney-shaped, smooth-surfaced leaves, found on furrowed petioles, can reach a width of 3 cm and a length of 15 cm. The leaf margin can be smooth, crenate, or slightly lobed. Usually three to six red flowers arise in a sessile manner or on very short pedicels in axillary umbels at the end of 2- –8-mm-long peduncles. The fruit, formed throughout the growing season, is approximately 5 mm long, with seven to nine ribs and a curved, strongly thickened pericarp.[1] The entire plant is used medicinally, with harvesting occurring at any time during the year.[1]

Chemical composition

Triterpenoid (steroid-like) compounds represent the primary pharmacological compounds in C. asiatica.[2] The chemical profile of Centella has been made difficult as a result of duplicate names and contradictory findings. In addition, sources of Centella from India, Sri Lanka, and Madagascar apparently do not contain the same constituents.[3,4] In India, at least three chemical races of C. asiatica are known.[5]

The concentration of triterpenes in gotu kola can vary 1.1–8%, with most samples yielding a concentration of 2.2–3.4%.[5] The major triterpenoid components of C. asiatica are asiatic acid, madecassic acid, asiaticoside, and madecassoside. The percentage of each tritepenoid in the Madagascar variety (the one most commonly used to produce standardized extracts) is as follows: asiatic acid (29–30%), madecassic acid (29–30%), asiaticoside (40%), and madecassoside (1–2%).[2]

Centella also contains a green, strongly volatile oil that contains an unidentified terpene acetate which accounts for 36% of the total oil, along with camphor, cineole, and other essential oils. Centella oil also contains glycerides of fatty acids; various plant sterols such as campesterol, stigmasterol, and sitosterol; and various polyacetylene compounds.[1,2]

Other notable compounds isolated from gotu kola include the flavonoids kaempferol, quercetin, and their glycosides; myoinositol; sugars; a bitter substance known as vellarin; amino acids; and resins.[1,2]

History and folk use

C. asiatica has been used as a medicine in India since prehistoric times. It is thought to be identical to the plant manduka parni, listed in the Susruta Samhita, an ancient Hindu text. Centella was also used extensively, both internally and externally, as a medicine by the people of Java and other islands of Indonesia. The medicinal use of this plant in India and Indonesia centered around its ability to heal wounds and relieve leprosy.[1]

In the 19th century, the plant and its extracts were incorporated into the Indian pharmacopeia where, in addition to being recommended for wound healing, it was recommended in the treatment of numerous skin conditions such as leprosy, lupus, varicose ulcers, eczema, and psoriasis; diarrhea; fever; amenorrhea; and diseases of the female genitourinary tract.[1]

In China, the leaves are prescribed for turbid menstrual discharge and toxic fevers, and the shoots are used for boils and fevers. The plant is also used in the treatment of fractures, contusions, strains, and snakebites.[1]

Centella was also used in China to delay aging. One of the reported "miracle elixers of life," its reputation as a promoter of longevity stems from the report of a Chinese herbalist, LiChing Yun, who allegedly lived 256 years. LiChing Yun's longevity was supposedly a result of his regular use of an herbal mixture chiefly composed of *Centella*.[6,7]

Extracts of *C. asiatica* were accepted as a drug in France during the 1880s. Since then, extracts have been used clinically in the treatment of many conditions. Gotu kola has aroused much curiosity from American consumers. Many consumers confuse gotu kola with kolanuts and assume gotu kola's rejuvenating activity is nothing more than an effect of caffeine. However, gotu kola is not related to the kolanut (*Cola nitida* or *C. acuminata*), nor does it contain any caffeine.

Pharmacology

C. asiatica, specifically the triterpenes, exerts remarkable wound-healing activity. Although the exact mechanism of action is not yet fully explained, a number of interesting observations have been made.

In one of the early pharmacological investigations of gotu kola, Boiteau and Ratsimamanga demonstrated that asiaticoside substantially hastened the healing process of experimentally induced wounds.[8] These authors concluded that asiaticoside works selectively in stimulating the rapid and healthy growth of the reticuloendothelial system.

Additional studies on the mechanisms of action of gotu kola in enhancing wound healing have shown that asiaticoside given orally, by intramuscular injection, or by implantation to rats, mice, guinea pigs, and rabbits produces the following effects:

1. Stimulates hair and nail growth[1,8,9,10]
2. Increases vascularization of connective tissue[1,8,9,10]
3. Increases the formation of mucin and structural components of connective tissues such as glycosaminoglycans, including hyaluronic acid and chondroitin sulfate[1,8,9,10,12]
4. Increases the tensile integrity of the dermis, the support structure of the skin[1,8,9,10]
5. Increases keratinization of the epidermis through stimulation of the stratum germinativum[1,10,12,13,14]
6. Possesses a eutrophic or balancing effect on connective tissue[1,10]

The outcome of gotu kola's complex actions is a balanced multiphasic effect on cells and tissues participating in the process of healing, particularly connective tissues. The development of a normal connective tissue matrix is perhaps the prime therapeutic action of *C. asiatica*.

It is obvious from the brief description of gotu kola's pharmacological activity that this plant is a valuable agent for the healing of wounds. An abridged list of additional therapeutic applications of *C. asiatica* follows. Several of the more popular uses of this valuable plant are discussed.

CLINICAL APPLICATIONS OF *C. ASIATICA*
USING EXTRACTS AND COMMERCIAL FORMULATIONS

Anal fissure[15]	Mental retardation[38]
Bladder ulcers[16,17]	Mycosis fungiodes[37]
Burns[18,19]	Peptic ulcer[39,40]
Cellulite[20-25]	Perineal lesions[41]
Cirrhosis[26-28]	Periodontal disease[42]
Dermatitis[20,29]	Retinal detachment[43]
Fibrocystic breast[30]	Scleroderma[44-47]
Hemorrhoids[31]	Skin ulcers[48-55]
Keloids[32-34]	Surgical wound[8,43,49,56-61]
Leprosy[11,19,35,36]	Tuberculosis[8,62]
Lupus erythematosus[37]	Venous disorders[63-75]

Burns

The standardized extract from *C. asiatica* has been used in the therapy of patients with second- and third-degree burns caused by various accidents (such as boiling water, electric current, and gas explosion).[18,19] Daily local application and/or intramuscular injections of the extract gave excellent results if the treatment was begun immediately after the accident. The extract prevented or limited the shrinking and swelling of the skin caused by skin infection and inhibited scar formation, increased healing, and decreased fibrosis.

Cellulite

Standardized extracts of *C. asiatica* have demonstrated good results in the treatment of cellulite in a number of clinical studies.[10,20-25] Bourguignon observed the action of the extract on several types of cellulite in 65 patients who had undergone other therapies without success. Over a period of 3 months, the extract produced very good results in 58% of the patients and satisfactory results in 20% of the patients.[20] Other investigations have shown a similar success rate (approximately 80%) in the treatment of cellulite.[21-24] The effect of gotu kola in the treatment of cellulite appears related to its ability to enhance connective tissue structure and reduce skin hardening.

Cirrhosis of the liver

Darnis et al. reported the therapeutic use of an extract of *C. asiatica* in alcohol-induced cirrhosis (six patients), cirrhosis of unknown etiology (two patients), and chronic hepatitis.[26] In the cirrhosis patients, an improvement in the histological findings and a regression of inflammatory infiltration was observed. No effect was observed in the patients with chronic hepatitis. Other reports have supported the use of gotu kola in fibrotic conditions of the liver.[27,28]

Keloids

The standardized extract of *Centella asiatica* has demonstrated impressive clinical results in the treatment of keloids and hypertrophic scars.[32-34] Its mechanism of action appears to be multifaceted but seems to result mainly from the reduction of the inflammatory phase of scar formation while simultaneously enhancing the maturation phase of scar formation.

Keloids and hypertrophic scars are characterized by a prolonged inflammatory phase that may go on for months or even years without progressing to maturation. The inflammatory phase is characterized histologically by high numbers of immature, swollen collagen bundles intermingled with inflammatory debris. The maturation phase is characterized by mature fibrocytes, normal collagen fibers, and few inflammatory cell elements.

In one study, a total of 227 patients with keloids or hypertrophic scars were treated with an orally administered, standardized *Centella* extract (effective dosage 60–90 mg). In the study, 139 patients used the extract alone (curative group), and 88 patients used the extract along with surgical scar revision (preventive group).[32] Among the curative group, 116 patients (82%) were found after 2–18 months to have benefited from the extract, either by relief of their symptoms or by disappearance of the inflammatory phase.

A double-blind study was conducted with 35 patients from the curative group. In this study, 22 out of 27 patients who received the extract improved. Nine of 19 patients given a placebo improved.

In the preventive group of 88 patients, the *Centella* extract also demonstrated significant positive effects. The therapeutic course in these patients was started a few weeks prior to surgery. If the researchers observed a positive response, the patient was brought to surgery and kept on the extract for 3 months. (This method of preselection allowed the researchers to offer other forms of therapy to unresponsive patients.) Clinical improvement was observed in 72 of the 88 patients (79%). This study highlights the therapeutic value of gotu kola in both preventing and reducing keloids.

Leprosy

Several investigators have reported impressive clinical results using C. asiatica and its extracts (orally, intramuscularly, and/or topically) in the treatment of leprosy in uncontrolled as well as controlled studies.[11,19,35,36] Therapeutic response is comparable to that of Dapsone, the standard drug used in the treatment of leprosy.

In addition to its wound-healing activity, it appears that asiaticoside (in an oxidized form, oxyasiaticoside) inhibits the growth of the tubercle bacillus in vitro and in vivo by dissolving the waxy coating of Mycobacterium leprae.[8]

Improving mental function

Appa Rao et al. reported a significant increase in the mental abilities of 30 developmentally disabled children treated with C. asiatica.[38] After a 12-week period, the children were more attentive and better able to concentrate on assigned tasks.

The triterpenes in gotu kola have demonstrated mild tranquilizing, anti-stress, and antianxiety action via enhancing cholinergic mechanisms.[77] Presumably, it is this enhancement of cholinergic mechanisms that is responsible for the effect in improving mental function as well.

Scleroderma

The standardized extract of C. asiatica has been tested in several trials for the treatment of scleroderma (including systemic sclerosis).[44-47] In addition to decreasing skin induration, the extract may lessen arthralgia and may improve motility of fingers. Presumably, the positive therapeutic response is a result of centella's eutrophic effect on connective tissue, thereby preventing the excessive collagen synthesis observed in scleroderma.

Venous disorders

Numerous studies have demonstrated that standardized extracts of C. asiatica are effective in the treatment of venous insufficiency as a result of enhancing the connective tissue structure of the perivascular sheath, reducing sclerosis or hardening, and improving the blood flow through the affected limbs.[1,10,63-75]

Researchers observed significant improvement in symptoms (feelings of heaviness in the lower legs, numbness, nighttime cramps, etc.), physical findings (swelling, spider veins, skin ulcers, vein distensibility, etc.), and functional capacity (improved venous blood flow) in approximately 80% of patients in the clinical trials.[1,10,63-75]

Wound healing

Many clinical studies have shown that standardized extracts of *C. asiatica* greatly aid wound repair.[1,8,10,43,48-61] The types of wounds healed include surgical wounds such as episiotomies and ENT surgeries; skin ulcers due to arterial or venous insufficiency; traumatic injuries to the skin; gangrene; skin grafts; schistosomiasis lesions; and perineal lesions produced during childbirth.

Summary

C. asiatica contains compounds that exert a balancing effect on connective tissue. The net effect is improved function and integrity of the collagen matrix and supportive structures. These effects are useful in the treatment of a wide range of conditions. The most popular therapeutic applications of gotu kola are in cases of varicose veins, cellulite, and wound repair.

Dosage

The majority of clinical studies on *C. asiatica* used standardized proprietary formulas available in Europe (e.g., Madecassol, TECA, and Centelase). These titrated extracts of *C. asiatica* contain asiaticoside (40%), asiatic acid (29–30%), madecassic acid (29–30%), and madecassoside (1–2%). The usual oral dosage of these formulas is 60–120 mg/day.

Because the concentration of triterpenes in gotu kola can vary from 1.1–8%, it is difficult to calculate an appropriate dosage when simply using the crude plant material. However, most samples yield a concentration of 2.2–3.4%. Therefore, about 2–4 g of crude plant material daily would contain an appropriate amount of triterpenes, although it is not known if this correlates with the clinical efficacy of the standardized extracts.

- Standardized extract containing asiaticoside (40%), asiatic acid (29 to 30%), madecassic acid (29 to 30%), and madecassoside (1 to 2%)—60–120 mg/day
- Crude dried plant leaves—2–4 g/day

- Tincture (1:5)—10–20 ml (1–2 tblsp)
- Fluid extract (1:1)—2.0–4.0 ml (½–1 tsp)

Toxicology

C. asiatica and its extracts are generally well tolerated. The clinical studies using the standardized extract of gotu kola indicate extremely good tolerance when administered orally.[1] The topical application of a salve containing gotu kola has been reported to cause contact dermatitis, although quite infrequently.[1]

Although the oral administration of asiaticoside at a dose of 1 g/kg body weight has not proved toxic in toxicology studies, the toxic dose of asiaticoside by intramuscular application to mice and rabbits is reported at 40–50 mg/kg body weight.[1]

Asiaticoside has been implicated as a possible carcinogen to the skin where repeated applications are used.[76] Teratological studies in which *C. asiatica* was administered to rabbits have proved negative.[32]

References

1. Kartnig T: Clinical applications of Centella asiatica (L.) Urb. Herbs Spices Medicinal Plants 3:146-73, 1988
2. Castellani C, Marai A and Vacchi P: The Centella asiatica. Boll Chim Farm 120:570-605, 1981
3. Battacharya SC: Constituents of Centella asiatica. I. Examination of the Ceylonese variety. J Ind Chem Soc 33:579-86, 1956
4. Battacharya SC: Constituents of Centella asiatica. I. Examination of the Indian variety. J Ind Chem Soc 33:893-8, 1956
5. Rao PS and Seshadri TR: Variation in the chemical composition of Indian samples of Centella asiatica. Curr Sci 38:77-9, 1969
6. Duke JA: Handbook of Medicinal Herbs. CRC Press, Boca Raton, FL 1985
7. Tyler V, Brady L and Robbers J: Pharmacognosy, 8th ed. Lea & Febiger, Philadelphia, PA 1981
8. Boiteau P and Ratsimamnga AR: Asiaticoside extracted from Centella asiatica, its therapeutic uses in the healing of experimental or refractory wounds, leprosy, skin tuberculosis, and lupus. Therapie 11:125-49, 1956
9. Boiteau P, Nigeon-Dureuil M and Ratsimamnga AR: Action of asiaticoside on reticuloendothelial tissue. Acad Sci Compt Rend 232:760-2, 1951
10. Monograph: Centella asiatica. Indena S.p.A., Milan, Italy, 1987
11. Abou-Chaar CI: New drugs from higher plants recently introduced into therapeutics. Lebanese Pharm J 8:15-37, 1963
12. Lawrence JC: The morphological and pharmacological effects of asiaticoside upon skin in vitro and in vivo. Europ J Pharmacol 1:414-24, 1967
13. Lawrence JC: The effect of asiaticoside on guinea pig skin. J Invest Dermatol 49:95-6, 1967
14. May A: The effect of asiaticoside on pig skin in organ culture. Europ J Pharmacol 4:177-81, 1968
15. Bensaude A: The treatment of anal fissure. Phleobologie 33:683-8, 1980
16. Aziz-Fam A: Use of titrated extract of Centella asiatica (TECA) in bilharzial bladder lesions. Int Surg 58:451-2, 1973
17. Etrebi A, Ibrahim A and Zaki K: Treatment of bladder ulcer with asiaticoside. J Egypt Med Assoc 58:324-7, 1975
18. Gravel JA: Oxygen dressings and asiaticoside in the treatment of burns. Laval Med 36:413-5, 1965

19. Boiteau P and Ratsimamanga AR: Important cicatrizants of vegetable origin and the biostimulins of Filatov. Bull Soc Sci Bretagne 34:307-15, 1959
20. Bourguignon D: Study of the action of titrated extract of Centella asiatica in chronic hepatic disorders. Sem Hosp Paris 55:1749-50, 1979
21. Bonnett GF: Treatment of localized cellulitis with asiaticoside Madecassol. Progr Med 102:109-10, 1974
22. Grosshans E and Keller F: Cellulite: reality or imposter? J Med Strasbourg 14:563-7, 1983
23. Keller F and Grosshans E: Cellulitis: reality or fraud? Med Hyg 41:1513-8, 1983
24. Tenailleau A: On 80 cases of cellulitis treated with the standard extract of Centella asiatica. Quest Med 31:919-24, 1978
25. Carraro Pereira I: Treatment of cellulitis with Centella asiatica. Folha Med 79:401-4, 1979
26. Darnis F, Orcel L, de Saint-Maur PP and Mamou P: Use of a titrated extract of Centella asiatica in chronic hepatic disorders. Sem Hosp Paris 55:1749-50, 1979
27. El Zawahry MD, Khalil AM and El Banna MH: Madecassol, a new therapy for hepatic fibrosis. Bull Soc Int Chir (Belgium) 34:296-7, 1975
28. El Zawahry MD, Khalil AM and El Banna MH: Madecassol, a new therapy for hepatic fibrosis. Bull Soc Int Chir (Belgium) 34:573-7, 1975
29. Fincato M: On the treatment of cutaneous lesions with extract of Centella asiatica. Minerva Chir 15:1235-8, 1960
30. Sterkers Desagnat M, Philbert M and Moreau L: Medical treatments for benign disease of the breast. Therapeutique 51:121-4, 1975
31. Guarnerio F, Sansonetti G, Donzelli R and Marelli C: Treatment of hemorrhoids with Centella asiatica. G Ital Angiol 6:46-52, 1986
32. Bosse JP, Papillon J, Frenette G, et al: Clinical study of a new antikeloid drug. Ann Plast Surg 3:13-21, 1979
33. Basset A, Ullmo A, Maleville J and Alt J: Treatment of keloids with Madecassol. Bull Soc Fr Dermatol Syph 77:826-7, 1970
34. Ipppolito F: Medical treatment of keloids. G Ital Dermatol 112:377-81, 1977
35. Chakrabarty T and Deshmukh S: Centella asiatica in the treatment of leprosy. Science Culture 42:573, 1976
36. Chudhuri S, Ghosh S, Chakrabarty T, Kundu S and Hazra SK: Use of a common Indian herb "Man-dukaparni" in the treatment of leprosy. J Ind Med Assoc 70:177-80, 1978
37. Wolram VS: Erfahrungern mit Maddecassol bei der behandlung ulzereroserser hautveranderungen. Wien Med Wschr 115:439-42, 1965
38. Appa Rao MVR, Srinivasan K and Koteswara RTL The effect of Centella asiatica on the general mental ability of mentally retarded children. Ind J Pschiatry 19:54-9, 1977
39. Kyoo WC: Medical treatment of peptic ulcer. J Korean Med Assoc 23:31-5, 1980
40. Pergola F: Treatment of peptic ulcer with a titrated extract of Centella asiatica. Med Chir Dig 36:445-8, 1974
41. Baudon-Glanddier B: Perineal lesions and asiaticoside. Gaz Med Fr 70:2463-4, 1963
42. Benedicenti A, Galli D and Merlini A: The clinical therapy of periodontal disease: the use of potassium hydroxide and the water-alcohol extract of Centella asiatica in combination with laser therapy in the treatment of severe periodontal disease. Parodontol Stomatol 24:11-26, 1985
43. Abou-Shousha ES and Khalil HA: Effect of asiaticoside (Madecassol) on the healing process in cataract surgical wounds and retinal detachment operations (clinical and experimental study). Bull Ophthalmol Soc Egypt 60:451-70, 1967
44. Bletry O: Comment on the treatment of scleroderma. Gazz Med Fr 87:1989-90, 1980
45. Fontan I, Rommel A, Geniaux M and Maleville J: Localized scleroderma. Concours Med 109:498-504, 1987
46. Sasaki S, Shinkai H, Akashi Y and Kishihara Y: Experimental and clinical effects of asiaticoside (Madecassol) on fibroblasts, granulomas, and scleroderma. Jap J Clin Dermatol 25:585-93, 1971
47. Sasaki S, Shinkai H, Akashi Y and Kishihara Y: Studies on the mechanism of action of asiaticoside (Madecassol) on experimental granulation tissue and cultured fibroblasts and its clinical application in systemic scleroderma. Acta Diabetol Lat 52:141-50, 1972
48. Balina LM, Cardama JE, Gatti JC, Ellis W and Wilkinson FF: Clinical results of an asiaticoside in cutaneous ulcerous lesions. Dia Med 33:1693-6, 1961
49. Bazex J, Nogue J and Peyrot J: Periulcerous eczema type cutaneous reaction during and after ulcers of the leg. Rev Med Toulouse 18:171-4, 1982
50. Dulauney MM: Posphlebitic leg ulcers and indications for therapy. Bordeaux Med 12:1807-10, 1979
51. Hanna LK, Amin L and El Serafy I: Trophic ulcers and their treatment with Madecassol. Afr Med 8:315-8, 1969

212

52. Huriez CL: Action of the titrated extract of Centella asiatica ub cicatrization of leg ulcers (10 - mg tablets). Apropos of 50 cases. Lille Med 17:suppl.3:574-9, 1972
53. Sarteel AM and Merlen JF: Treatment of leg ulcers. Phlebologie 36:375-9, 1983
54. Thiers H, Fayolle J, Boiteau P and Ratsimamanga AR: Asiaticoside, the active principle of Centella asiatica, in the treatment of cutaneous ulcers. Lyon Med 197:389-85, 1957
55. Vittori F: The treatment of ulcus cruris. J Med Lyon 63:429-32, 1982
56. Castellani C, Gillet JY, Lavernhe G and Dellenbach P: Asiaticoside and cicatrization of episiotomies. Bull Fed Soc Gynecol Obstet 18:184-6, 1966
57. Collonna d'Istria J: Research on the healing action of Madecassol in cervical and laryngeal surgery after ionizing radiations. J Fr Otorhinolaryngol 19:507-10, 1970
58. O'Keeffe P: A trial of asiaticoside on skin graft donor areas. Brit J Plast Surg 27:194-5, 1974
59. Pignataro O and Teatini GP: Clinical research on the cicatrizing action of Madecassol in comparison of oropharyngeal mucosa. Minerva Med 56:2683-6, 1965
60. Riu R, Alavoine J, Auriault A and Le Mouel C: Clinical study of Madecassol in otorhinology. J Med Lyon 47:693-706, 1966
61. Sevin P: Some observations on the use of asiaticoside (Madecassol) in general surgery. Progr Med (France) 90:23-4, 1962
62. King DS: Tuberculosis. New Engl J Med 243:530-6, 565-71, 1950
63. Allegra C: Comparative capillaroscopic study of certain bioflavonoids and total triterpenic fractions of Centella asiatica in venous insufficiency. Clin Terap 110:550- 1984
64. Allegra C, Pollari G, Criscuolo A, et al: Centella asiatica extract in venous disorders of the lower limbs. Comparative clinico-instrumental studies with a placebo. Clin Terap 99:507-13, 1981
65. Barletta S, Borgioli A and Corsi C: Results with Centella asiatica in chronic venous insufficiency. Gazz Med Ital 140:33-5, 1981
66. Basellini A, Agus GB, Antonucci E and Papacharalambus D: Varicose disease in pregnancy. Ann Ostet Ginecol Med Perinat 106:337-41, 1985
67. Boely C: Indications of titrated extract of Centella asiatica in phlebology. Gazz Med Fr 82:741-4, 1975
68. Bolgert M and Gautron G: An extract from Centella asiatica in phlebology. Progr Med (France) 100:31-2, 1972
69. Cappelli R: Clinical and pharmacological study on the effect of an extract of Centella asiatica in chronic venous insufficiency of lower limbs. G Ital Angiol 3:44-8, 1983
70. Cospite M, Ferrara F, Milio G and Meli F: Study about pharmacologic and clinical activity of Centella asiatica titrated extract in the chronic venous deficiency of the lower limbs: valuation with strain gauge phlethismography. G Ital Angiol 4:200-5, 1984
71. Frausini G, Rotatori T and Oliva S: Controlled trial on clinical-dynamic effects of three treatments in chronic venous insufficiency. G Ital Angiol 5:147-51, 1985
72. Marastoni F, Baldo A, Redaelli G, and Ghiringhelli L: Centella asiatica extract in venous pathology of the lower limbs and its evaluation as compared with tribenoside. Minerva-Cardioangiol 30:201-7, 1982
73. Mariani G and Patuzzo E: Treatment of venous insufficiency with extract of Centella asiatica. Clin Eur (Italy) 22:154-8, 1983
74. Mazzola C and Gini MM: Centella asiatica extract in treatment of chronic venous insufficiency. Clin Eur (Italy) 21:160-6 1982
75. Pointel JP, Boccalon H, Cloarec M, et al: Titrated extract of Centella asiatica (TECA) in the treatment of venous insufficiency of the lower limbs. Angiology 38:46-50, 1987
76. Laerum OD and Iversen OH: Reticuloses and epidermal tumors in hairless mice after topical skin applications of cantharidin and asiaticoside. Cancer Research 32:1463-9, 1972
77. Ramaswamy AS, Periyasamy SM and Basu N: Pharmacological studies on Centella asiatica Linn (Brahma manduki) (N.O. Umbelliferae. Jour Res Ind Med 4:160-75, 1970

29

Sarsaparilla

(SMILAX SARSAPARILLA)

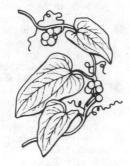

Key uses of sarsaparilla:

- Psoriasis
- Eczema
- General tonic

General description

Sarsaparilla is a tropical American perennial plant. Its long, slender root and short, thick rhizomes produce a vine that trails on the ground and climbs by means of tendrils growing in pairs from the petioles of the alternate, obicular to ovate, evergreen leaves. The root is the part of the plant utilized for medicinal purposes.

Chemical composition

Sarsaparilla contains 1.8–2.4% steroid saponins, including sarsaponin, smilasaponin, sarsaparilloside, and its aglycones sarsapogenin, smilagenin, pollinastanol. Other constituents include starch, resins, and a trace of volatile oil.[1]

History and folk use

Sarsaparilla's medicinal use has been as a tonic and a blood purifier. Tonics are defined as agents that "permanently exalt the energies of the body at large, without vitally affecting any one organ in particular."[2] In short, tonics tone the whole system.

A blood purifier, or depurative, refers to an agent that cleanses and purifies the system.[2] Sarsaparilla's reputation in this regard probably stems from its use in the treatment of syphilis during the 16th century. It was imported at that time from the Caribbean and South America to Europe.

A French physician, Nicholas Monardes, published a comprehensive account of sarsaparilla and several other "new" drugs in the treatment of syphilis in 1574. Many Europeans at the time believed that syphilis had come to Europe from the West Indies with Columbus' sailors. Because sarsaparilla came from the same region in which syphilis was presumed to have originated, physicians held much hope for this new herbal remedy.

Sarsaparilla was a welcome alternative to mercury, the standard treatment of syphilis (a treatment that often caused more deaths than the disease itself). Sarsaparilla was also used by the Chinese in the treatment of syphilis. Clinical observations in China demonstrated that sarsaparilla is effective, according to blood tests, in about 90% of acute cases and 50% of chronic cases.[1,4] Sarsaparilla species have been used all over the world in many different cultures for the same conditions—namely gout, arthritis, fevers, digestive disorders, skin disease, and cancer.[1]

Pharmacology

The mechanism of action of sarsaparilla is largely unknown, although the plant does contain several saponins and has been shown to be clinically effective in the treatment of psoriasis.[1,5,6] This evidence points to a possible effect on the binding of cholesterol and bacterial toxins in the intestines.

Endotoxin binding

Evidence seems to support sarsaparilla as an endotoxin binder. Endotoxins are cell wall constituents of bacteria that are absorbed from the gut. Normally, the liver plays a vital role by filtering these and other gut-derived compounds before they reach the general circulation. If the amount of endotoxin absorbed is excessive, or if the liver is not functioning adequately, the liver can become overwhelmed and endotoxins will spill into the blood.[7]

If endotoxins are allowed to circulate, the alternate complement system is activated. This system plays a critical role in aggravating inflammatory processes, and activation of complement is responsible for much of the inflammation and cell damage that occurs in many diseases, including gout, arthritis, and psoriasis.[7] These conditions have been treated throughout history by sarsaparilla.

Individuals with psoriasis have been shown to have high levels of circulating endotoxins. Binding of endotoxin in the intestines is associated with clinical improvement in these individuals. In a controlled study of 92 patients, an endotoxin-binding saponin (sarsaponin) from sarsaparilla greatly improved the psoriasis in 62% of the patients and resulted in complete clearance in 18%.[6]

Further support of sarsaparilla's effect as a binder of endotoxin is its historical use in the treatment of fever. (Absorbed endotoxins produce fever.[7]) Sarsaparilla also exhibits some antibiotic activity, but this is probably secondary to its endotoxin-binding action.[1]

Tonic and blood purifier

Despite sarsaparilla's long history of use, there is little scientific information on this plant. From the limited information available, it appears that sarsaparilla's medicinal effects are a result of components binding bacterial endotoxins in the gut in a way that renders them unabsorbable. This factor greatly reduces the stress on the liver and other organs and is probably responsible for sarsaparilla's historical use as a tonic and blood purifier. This ability to bind endotoxins is probably why sarsaparilla is reported to be effective in many cases of psoriasis, gout, and arthritis.

Sarsaparilla and the testosterone controversy

Sarsparilla has been widely touted as a "sexual rejuvenator." Some commercial suppliers have even claimed that it is a rich source of human testosterone. The fact is, sarsaparilla may have good tonic effects, but there is no actual testosterone in the plant. It is unlikely that the steroid-like substances in sarsaparilla are absorbed to any great degree. It is also unlikely that sarsaparilla has any significant anabolic effects because there is no evidence to support that it increases muscle mass. Laboratory experiments have demonstrated that the sarsaparilla saponin, sarsasapgenin, can be synthetically transformed to testosterone. However, it is extremely unlikely that this reaction could take place in the human body. These data contribute to the confusion over sarsaparilla as a "sexual rejuvenator."

Summary

Sarsaparilla contains saponins, or steroid-like molecules, that bind to intestine endotoxins. This effect may support the plant's historical use as a blood purifier and a tonic. These effects may be of benefit in human health conditions associated with high endotoxin levels, most notably, psoriasis, eczema, arthritis, and ulcerative colitis.

Dosage

Three times a day dosages:

- Dried root—1–4 g or by decoction
- Liquid extract (1:1)—8–16 ml (2–4 tsp)
- Solid extract (4:1)—250 mg

Toxicology

Although no adverse effects from the use of sarsaparilla have been reported, it is possible that problems could arise if large doses were used over a long period of time.

References

1. Leung AY: Encyclopedia of Common Natural Ingredients Used in Food, Drugs and Cosmetics. John Wiley & Sons, New York, NY, 1980
2. Felter HW: The Eclectic Materia Medica, Pharmacology and Therapeutics. Eclectic Medical Publications, Portland, OR, 1983
3. Griggs B: Green Pharmacy, A History of Herbal Medicine. Jill Norman & Hobhouse. London, 1981
4. Bensky D and Gamble A: Chinese Herbal Medicine Materia Medica. Eastland Press, Seattle, WA, 1986
5. Duke JA: Handbook of Medicinal Herbs. CRC Press, Boca Raton, FL 1985
6. Thurman FM: The treatment of psoriasis with sarsaparilla compound. NEJM 227:128-33, 1942
7. Pizzorno JE and Murray MT: A Textbook of Natural Medicine. JBC Publications, Seattle, WA. 1987 pp. Chapter IV:Alternate Complement Pathway and Chapter IV:Bowel Toxemia

30

Australian tea tree

(MELALEUCA ALTERNIFOLIA)

Key uses of tea tree oil:

- Topical antiseptic
- Athlete's foot
- Boils
- Wound healing

General description

Melaleuca alternifolia, or tea tree, is a small tree native to only one area of the world—the northeast coastal region of New South Wales, Australia. The leaves are the portion of the plant that is used medicinally. The leaves are the source of a valuable therapeutic oil, tea tree oil. Although there are over 50 members of the Melaleuca family, only the oil from *M. alternifolia* is the true tea tree oil with therapeutic qualities.

Chemical composition

Tea tree leaves contain about 1.8% of an oil.[1] It is the tea tree oil that is of chief medical interest. This oil contains over 48 compounds but is chiefly composed of 1,8-cineol, gamma-terpinene, *p*-cymene and 1-terpinen-4-ol, and other terpenes.[2] The Australian Standard (AS 2782-1985) for oil of Melaleuca (terpinen-4-ol type) sets a minimum content of terpinen-4-ol at 30% and a maximum 1,8-cineol content of 15%.[1]

History and folk use

The medicinal properties of crushed tea tree leaves were known to the Bundjabug Aborigines of northern New South Wales. In fact, the waters of the lagoon where tea tree leaves had fallen and decayed for hundreds of years were viewed as having tremendous healing properties.[1]

The popular name of tea tree was first reported in Captain Cook's account of his second voyage, titled *A Voyage to the South Pole*, in 1777:

> We at first made it (some beer) of a decoction of the spruce leaves; but finding that this alone made the beer too astringent, we afterwards mixed with it an equal quantity of the tea plant (a name it obtained in my former voyage from our using it as tea then, as we also did now), which partly destroyed the astringency of the other, and made the beer exceedingly palatable, and esteemed by everyone on board.[1]

The early settlers of Australia use the leaves of *M. alternifolia* to make tea, hence the further use of the popular name of tea tree.[1]

The medical world's first mention of tea tree appeared in the *Medical Journal of Australian* in 1930.[3] A surgeon in Sydney reported some impressive results using a solution of tea tree oil for cleaning surgical wounds:

> The results obtained in a variety of conditions when it (tea tree oil) was first tried were most encouraging, a striking feature being that it dissolved pus and left the surface of infected wounds clean so that its germicidal action become more effective without any apparent damage to the tissues. This was something new, as most efficient germicides destroy tissue as well as bacteria.

Other favorable reports followed in the early 1930s. During World War II, tea tree oil was used as a disinfectant and actually issued to soldiers. The Australian Army commandeered supplies of the oil and exempted leaf cutters from national service in order to maintain production. The production of tea tree oil during World War II was regarded as an essential industry.[1]

After World War II, the tea tree oil industry stagnated for more than 30 years, for a number of reasons, including the general trend away from natural products toward more highly valued synthetic chemicals. During the late 1970s and early 1980s the Australian tea tree oil industry was reborn, and successful plantations growing *M. alternifolia* were developed. The large-scale production of tea tree oil involves the use of technology to produce a consistently high quality oil.[1]

Pharmacology

Tea tree oil possesses significant antiseptic properties and is regarded by many as the ideal skin disinfectant. It is active against a wide range of organisms, penetrates the skin easily, and is nonirritating to the skin.[1] Organisms inhibited by tea tree oil include *Candida albicans, Staphylococcus aureus, Pseudomonas aeruginosa, Propionibacterium acnes, Streptococcus pyrogenes,* and *Trichophyon mentagrophytes.*[1]

Therapeutic uses of tea tree oil are based largely on its antiseptic and antifungal properties. Tea tree oil has been used in the following conditions: acne, apthous stomatitis (canker sores), athlete's foot, boils, burns, carbuncles, corns, empyema, gingivitis, herpes, impetigo, infections of the nail bed, insect bites, lice, mouth ulcers, psoriasis, root canal treatment, ringworm, sinus infections, sore throat, skin and vaginal infections, tinea, thrush, and tonsilitis.[1] A variety of tea tree oil-based products exist on the marketplace, including toothpastes, shampoos and conditioners, creams, hand and body lotions, soaps, gels, liniments, and nail polish removers.

Summary

Tea tree oil is an effective topical antiseptic that can be used to reduce microbial counts in a particular area, such as wounds, surgical incisions, and skin infections. A number of products in the marketplace contain tea tree oil. When using these products, simply follow the directions on the label. In addition, tea tree leaves can be used to make teas that may be of benefit in treating sore throat, tonsilitis, sinus infections, and colitis.

Toxicology

Tea tree oil is extremely safe to use as a topical antiseptic. However, the oral ingestion of tea tree oil cannot be recommended because it can be quite toxic. Tea made from the leaves of the tea tree can be ingested, however. Such tea is extremely safe and nontoxic.

References

1. Altman PM: Australian tea tree oil. Australian J Pharmacy 69:276-8, 1988
2. Swords G and Hunter GLK: Composition of Australian tea tree oil (Melaleuca alternifolia). J Agric Food Chem 26:3, 1978
3. Essential Oils Data Search Inc: Melaleuca alternifolia, a compilation of articles and papers about Australian tea tree oil. Vancouver, WA 1985

SECTION XII

An herb for the eyes

For normal vision to occur, light must interact with the specialized nerve cells of the eye (rods and cones) to create a nerve impulse. The nerve impulse is then transmitted to the visual areas of the brain. Many nutritional compounds are important in vision, both in terms of protecting the eye from damage as well as in the actual process of vision.

When normal protective mechanisms of the eye begin to fail as a result of aging, a variety of disorders develop, including glaucoma, cataracts, and macular degeneration. Every effort should be made to prevent these conditions from developing. This can be done by enhancing the health of the eye. The health of the eye is largely dependent on a rich supply of nutrients and oxygen. Relatively speaking, the amount of blood flow through the eye is the greatest in the body. This fact highlights the importance of nutrition for optimal eye health and function.

Bilberries (European blueberries) as well as other richly colored berries offer a broad range of important nutritional compounds to nourish the eye as well as to enhance visual function and prevent damage to important structures. Of great importance are a class of bioflavonoids found in bilberries and known as anthocyanosides. Anthocyanoside extract has many other uses in addition to treating eye complaints. These uses are fully described in the next chapter.

31

Bilberry
(VACCINIUM MYRTILLUS)

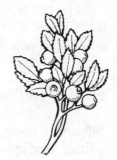

Key uses of bilberry:

- Diabetic retinopathy
- Macular degeneration
- Cataract
- Glaucoma
- Varicose veins

General description

There are 200 species in the Vaccinium family, most of which are found in the Northern Hemisphere. This chapter focuses on *Vaccinium myrtillus* (bilberry, huckleberry, or blueberry) and the medicinal use of extracts of its fruit.

V. myrtillus, or bilberry, is a shrubby perennial plant that grows in the sandy areas of the northern United States and in the woods and forest meadows of Europe. The angular, green, branched stem grows from a creeping rootstock to a height of 1–1.5 ft. The leaves are 0.5–1.0 in. long, oval, slightly dentate, and bright green. The flowers are reddish- or greenish-pink and bell-shaped. The flowering season is April–June. The fruit is a blue-black berry.[1]

Chemical composition

The active components of bilberries are its flavonoids, specifically its anthocyanosides. Other members of the Vaccinium family, including *Ribes nigum* (black currant) and *Vitis vinifera* (grape), contain similar anthocyanosides.[3] Extracts of these fruit, like bilberries, are also used for medicinal purposes in Europe.

The concentration of anthocyanosides in the fresh fruit is approximately 0.1–0.25%. Concentrated extracts of *V. myrtillus* yield an anthocyanoside content of nearly 40%.[2]

History and folk use

Bilberries have, of course, been used as food and for their high nutritive value. Medicinally, they have been used in the treatment of scurvy and urinary complaints (including infection and stones).[1] The dried berries have been used primarily for their astringent qualities in the treatment of diarrhea and dysentery. Decoctions of the leaves have been used in the treatment of diabetes.[1]

Pharmacology

The pharmacology of *V. myrtillus* will be discussed almost entirely in relationship to its anthocyanoside content because this has been the focus of research on this plant.

Collagen-stabilizing action

Anthocyanosides possess significant collagen-stabilizing action.[4-10] Collagen, the most abundant protein of the body, is responsible for maintaining the integrity of "ground substance" as well as tendons, ligaments, and cartilage. Collagen is destroyed during the inflammatory processes that occur in rheumatoid arthritis, periodontal disease, and other inflammatory conditions involving bones, joints, cartilage, and other connective tissue.

Anthocyanidins, proanthocyanidins, and other flavonoids are remarkable in their ability to prevent collagen destruction. The anthocyanidins in *V. myrtillus* extracts have been shown to affect collagen metabolism in several ways:

1. Anthocyanosides have the ability to actually crosslink collagen fibers, resulting in reinforcement of the natural crosslinking of collagen that forms the collagen matrix of connective tissue (ground substance, cartilage, tendon, etc.).[4-7,14]

2. Anthocyanosides prevent free radical damage with their potent anti-oxidant and free radical scavenging action.[4-8]

3. Anthocyanosides inhibit enzymatic cleavage of collagen by enzymes secreted by leukocytes during inflammation.[4-6,8,13,14]

4. Anthocyanosides and other flavonoid components of *V. myrtillus* prevent the release and synthesis of compounds that promote inflammation, such as histamine, serine proteases, prostaglandins, and leukotrienes.[4-6,11,12]

5. Anthocyanosides promote collagen synthesis as well as the synthesis of other ground substance components.[9,10,15]

Normalization of capillary permeability
and use in varicose veins

Anthocyanosides have strong "vitamin P" activity.[4] Included in their effects are an ability to increase vitamin C levels within cells and decrease capillary permeability and fragility.[4-6] Their effect in reducing capillary fragility and permeability is roughly twice that of the flavonoid rutin, both in terms of intensity and duration of action.[18]

V. myrtillus extracts have been widely used in Europe in the treatment of various arterial, venous, and capillary disorders. Clinical studies have demonstrated a positive effect in the treatment of capillary fragility, blood purpuras, various disturbances of blood flow to the brain (effects similar to those produced by *Ginkgo biloba*), venous insufficiency, varicose veins, and blood in the urine not caused by infection.[19-24,53-56]

Bilberry's effect in the treatment of a variety of disorders of veins relates to the ability of anthocyanosides to protect altered veins, like varicose veins, via two mechanisms: (1) increasing the barrier effect of the vein wall through stabilization of the cell membrane structures, and (2) increasing the biosynthesis of the components of the connective ground substance.[15]

One interesting effect of the normalization of collagen structures and capillaries is that anthocyanosides from *V. myrtillus* decreases the permeability of the blood brain barrier.[14,17] This barrier prevents large toxic molecules from entering the brain. Increased blood brain permeability has been linked to autoimmune diseases of the central nervous system, schizophrenia, "cerebral allergies," and a variety of other brain disorders. Presumably, the anthocyanosides inhibit destruction of the ground substance collagen of brain capillaries, thus helping maintain or restore the brain's protection from drugs, pollutants, naturally occurring toxins, and other brain toxins.[7,8,13,14,17]

Antiaggregation effect on platelets

Anthocyanosides, like many other flavonoids, have been shown to possess significant antiaggregation effects on platelets.[26-28] Excessive platelet aggregation is associated with an increased risk of heart attack and stroke.

Smooth muscle relaxing activity

Anthocyanoside extracts have demonstrated significant vascular smooth muscle-relaxing effects in a variety of experimental models.[29-31] The practical application of this research may be in the treatment of dysmenorrhea, for which a preliminary study has demonstrated positive effects.[32]

Ophthalmological applications

Perhaps the most significant therapeutic applications for *V. myrtillus* extracts are in the field of ophthalmology. Interest in anthocyanosides from this plant was first aroused when researchers observed that administering bilberry extracts to healthy subjects resulted in improved nighttime visual acuity, quicker adjustment to darkness, and faster restoration of visual acuity after exposure to glare.[33,34] Further studies confirmed these results.[35-38] Results were most impressive in individuals with retinitis pigmentosa and hemeralopia ("day blindness," or an inability to see distinctly in bright light).

It appears that anthocyanosides from *V. myrtillus* have an affinity for the pigmented epithelium of the retina, which composes the optical or functional part of the retina.[39] This is consistent with several of the clinical effects observed. Anthocyanoside extracts of this plant appear to be of great value in both poor night vision and poor day vision.

Glaucoma

V. myrtillus may play a significant role in the prevention and treatment of glaucoma via its effect on collagen structures in the eye. Collagen provides tensile strength and integrity to the tissues of the eye. Structural changes in the collagen of the eye precede clinically detectable abnormalities. These changes may result in elevated intraocular pressure (IOP) readings, the hallmark symptom of glaucoma, or, perhaps more significantly, the progression of peripheral vision loss. Changes in collagen structure would explain why there is similar peripheral vision loss in patients with normal and elevated IOP.

Therefore, primary prevention of glaucoma involves maintaining ground substance and collagen framework integrity. It is important to prevent the breakdown of collagen matrix as it is in other conditions involving collagen abnormalities (i.e., atherosclerosis, rheumatoid arthritis, and periodontal disease).

V. myrtillus consumption may offer significant protection against the development of glaucoma because of its collagen-enhancing actions. In addition, anthocyanosides may be of benefit in the treatment of chronic glaucoma because rutin has been demonstrated to lower IOP when used as an adjunct in patients unresponsive to miotics alone.[40] As stated, *V. myrtillus* anthocyanosides are much more biologically active than rutin.[18]

Cataracts and retinal degeneration

V. myrtillus anthocyanosides may offer significant protection against the development of retinal (macular) degeneration and cataracts, particularly diabetic retinopathy and diabetic cataracts. Both the rate of retinal degeneration[41] and the occurrence of cataracts[42] in rats has been retarded by changing their diet from a commercial "lab chow" to a "well-defined diet." Preliminary research suggests that flavonoid components in the well-defined diets may be responsible for the protective effects against cataracts and retinal degeneration.[10]

V. myrtillus anthocyanoside extracts are widely used in Europe in the prevention of diabetic retinopathy.[44-46] The positive effect noted in clinical trials may be the result of improved capillary integrity as well as inhibition of several factors responsible for damage to the eyes in diabetes.[47-49]

Diabetes mellitus

A decoction of blueberry leaves has a long history of folk use in the treatment of diabetes. This use is supported by research in which oral administration reduced elevated blood sugar levels in normal and depancreatized dogs, even when glucose was concurrently injected intravenously.[46,50]

The anthocyanoside myrtillin is apparently the most active blood sugar lowering component of *V. myrtillus*. Upon injection, it is somewhat weaker than insulin, but it is also less toxic, even at 50 times the 1 g/day therapeutic dose. A single dose can produce beneficial effects lasting for several weeks.[46]

The most important benefits from the use of anthocyanosides in the treatment of diabetes, however, relate to their ability to improve collagen integrity and capillary permeability. Benefit also may derive from the ability of the anthocyanaosides to inhibit sorbitol accumulation, thus providing protection from the serious vascular and neurological sequelae of diabetes.

V. myrtillus anthocyanosides have also been shown to have a protective effect on capillary fragility in diabetics and to reduce serum cholesterol and triglyceride levels in patients with elevated levels.[51] Although studies in rabbits have not confirmed a cholesterol-lowering effect, the anthocyanosides were able to significantly decrease the development of atherosclerosis. Presumably, this is a result of increasing collagen crosslinking, thus reducing the likelihood of fat and cholesterol being deposited in the artery.[52]

Inflammatory joint disease

The effects of anthocyanosides on collagen structures and their potent antioxidant activity make *V. myrtillus* anthocyanoside extracts extremely useful in the treatment of a wide variety of inflammatory conditions—most notably, rheumatoid arthritis. Bioflavonoids have been found to increase collagen synthesis and inhibit collagen catabolism in rats that have adjuvant-induced arthritis (a chronic progressive arthritis with some similarities to rheumatoid arthritis).[9]

Blueberries, like cherries,[16] are particularly valuable in the treatment of gout, a form of athritis. Their flavonoid components are able to reduce both uric acid levels and tissue destruction.

Summary

V. myrtillus anthocyanosides have exhibited significant pharmacological activity, particularly on collagen structures. Research has demonstrated a positive effect in the treatment of capillary fragility, blood purpuras, various encephalic circulation disturbances, venous insufficiency, varicose veins, poor night vision, day-blindness, and diabetic retinopathy.

Experimental studies indicate that anthocyanoside should be useful in most inflammatory or degenerative conditions involving connective tissues (e.g., osteoarthritis, gout, rheumatoid arthritis, periodontal disease), glaucoma, diabetes, cataracts, retinal degeneration, and possibly schizophrenia.

Dosage

The standard dose for *V. myrtillus* should be based on its anthocyanoside content, as calculated by its anthocyanidin percentage. Widely used pharmaceutical preparations in Europe are standardized for anthocyanidin content (typically 25%). Dosages of three times a day are as follows:

- Anthocyanosides (calculated as anthocyanidin)—20–40 mg
- *Vaccinium myrtillus* extract (25% anthocyanidin content)—80–160 mg
- Fresh berries—4–8 oz

Toxicology

Extensive investigation has demonstrated that *V. myrtillus* anthocyanoside extracts are without toxic effects. Administering doses as high as 400 mg/kg produced no apparent side effects in rats. Excess levels of anthocyanoside are quickly excreted through the urine and bile.[18,25]

References

1. Grieve M: A Modern Herbal, volume 1. Dover Publications, New York, NY, 1971, pp385-6
2. Baj A, Bombardelli E, Gabetta B, and Martinelli EM: Qualitative and quantitative evaluation of Vaccinium myrtillus anthocyanins by high-resolution gas chromatography and high-performance liquid chromatography. J Chromatogr 279:365-72, 1983
3. Andersen OM: Anthocyanins in fruits of Vaccinium uliginosum L. (bog whortleberry). J Food Sci 52:665-6,680, 1987
4. Kuhnau J: The flavonoids: A class of semi-essential food components: Their role in human nutrition. Wld Rev Nutr Diet 24:117-91, 1976
5. Gabor M: Pharmacologic effects of flavonoids on blood vessels. Angiologica 9:355-74, 1972
6. Havsteen B: Flavonoids, a class of natural products of high pharmacological potency. Biochem Pharmacol 32:1141-8, 1983
7. Monboisse JC, Braquet P, Randoux A, and Borel JP: Non-enzymatic degradation of acid-soluble calf skin collagen by superoxide ion: Protective effect of flavonoids. Biochem Pharmacol 32:53-8, 1983
8. Monboisse JC, Braquet P and Borel JP: Oxygen-free radicals as mediators of collagen breakage. Agents Actions 15:49-50, 1984
9. Rao CN, Rao VH and Steinman B: Influence of bioflavonoids on the collagen metabolism in rats with adjuvant induced arthritis. Ital J Biochem 30:54-62, 1981
10. Ronziere MC, Herbage D, Garrone R, and Frey J: Influence of some flavonoids on reticulation of collagen fibrils in vitro. Biochem Pharmacol 30:1771-6, 1981
11. Middleton E: The flavonoids. Trends in Phramaceutical Science 5:335-8, 1984
12. Amella M, Bronner C, Briancon F, et al: Inhibition of mast cell histamine release by flavonoids and biflavonoids. Planta Medica 51:16-20, 1985
13. Jonadet M, Meunier MT, Bastide J, and Bastide P: Anthocyanosides extracted from Vitis vinifera, Vaccinium myrtillus and Pinus maritimus. I. Elastase-inhibiting activities in vitro. II. Compared angio-protective activities in vivo. J Pharm Belg 38:41-6, 1983
14. Detre A, Jellinek H, Miskulin M, and Robert AM: Studies on vascular permeability in hypertension: action of anthocyanosides. Clin Physiol Biochem 4:143-9, 1986
15. Mian E, Curri SB, Lieti A, and Bombardelli E: Anthocyanosides and the walls of the microvessels: further aspects of the mechanism of action of their protective effect in syndromes due to abnormal capillary fragility. Minerva Med 68:3565-81, 1977
16. Blau LW: Cherry diet control for gout and arthritis. Tex Rep Biol Med 8:309-11, 1950
17. Robert AM, Godeau G, Moati F, and Miskulin M: Action of the anthocyanosides of Vaccinium myrtillus on the permeability of the blood brain barrier. J Med 8:321-32, 1977
18. Lietti A and Forni G: Studies on Vaccinium myrtillus anthocyanosides. I. Vasoprotective and anti-inflammatory activity. Arzneim Forsch 26:829-32, 1976
19. Ghiringhelli C, Gregoratti F and Marastoni F: Capillarotropic activity of anthocyanosides in high doses in phlebopathic stasis. Min Cardioangiol 26:255-76, 1978
20. Treviso A: Therapeutic value of the association of anthocyanin glucosides with glutamine and phosphorylserine in the treatment of learning disturbances at different ages. Gazz Med Ital 138:217-32, 1979
21. Grismond GL: Treatment of pregnancy-induced phlebopathies. Minerva Ginecol 33:221-30, 1981
22. Piovella F, Almasio P, Ricetti MM, Trpin L, and Cavanna L: Results with anthocyanidins in the treatment of haemorrhagic diathesis due to defective primary haemastasis. Gazz Med Ital 140:445-9, 1981
23. Pennarola R, Roco P, Matarazzo G, et al: The therapeutic action of the anthocyanosides in microcirculatory changes due to adhesive-induced polyneuritis. Gazz Med Ital 139:485-91, 1980
24. Amouretti M: Therapeutic value of Vaccinium myrtillus anthocyanosides in an internal medicine department. Therapeutique 48:579-81, 1972

25. Lietti A and Forni G: Studies on Vaccinium myrtillus anthocyanosides. II. Aspects of anthocyanins pharmacokinetics in the rat. Arzneim Forsch 26:832-5, 1976
26. Zaragoza F, Iglesias I and Benedi J: Comparison of thrombocyte antiaggregant effects of anthocyanosides with those of other agents. Arch Pharmacol Toxicol 11:183-8, 1985
27. Morazzoni P and Magistretti MJ: Effects of Vaccinium myrtillus anthocyanosides on prostacyclin like activity in rat arterial tissue. Fitoterapia 57:11-4, 1986
28. Bottecchia D, Bettini V, Martino R, and Camerra G: Preliminary report on the inhibitory effect of Vaccinium myrtillus anthocyanosides on platelet aggregation and clot retraction. Fitoterapia 48:3-8, 1987
29. Bettini V, Mavellaro F, Ton P, and Zanella P: Effects of Vaccinium myrtillus anthocyanosides on vascular smooth muscle. Fitoterapia 55:265-72, 1984
30. Bettini V, Mavellaro F, Patron E, et al: Inhibition by Vaccinium myrtillus anthocyanosides of barium-induced contractions in segments of internal thoracic vein. Fitoterapia 55:323-7, 1984
31. Bettini V, Mayellaro F, Pilla I, et al: Mechanical responses of isolated coronary arteries to barium in the presence of Vaccinium myrtillus anthocyanosides. Fitoterapia 56:3-10, 1985
32. Colombo D and Vescovini R: Controlled clinical trial of anthocyanosides from Vaccinium myrtillus in primary dysmenorrhea. G Ital Obstet Ginecol 7:1033-8, 1985
33. Jayle GE and Aubert L: Action des glucosides d'anthocyanes sur la vision scotopique et mesopique du sujet normal. Therapie 19:171-85,1964
34. Terrasse J and Moinade S: Premiers resultats obtenus avec un nouveau facteur vitamininique P "les anthocyanosides" extraits du Vaccinium myrtillus. Presse Med 72:397-400, 1964
35. Sala D, Rolando M, Rossi PL, and Pissarello L: Effect of anthocyanosides on visual performances at low illumination. Minerva Oftalmol 21:283-5, 1979
36. Gloria E and Peria A: Effect of anthocyanosides on the absolute visual threshold. Ann Ottalmol Clin Ocul 92:595-607, 1066
37. Junemann G: On the effect of anthocyanosides on hemeralopia following quinine poisoning. Klin Monatsbl Augenheilkd 151:891-6, 1967
38. Caselli L: Clinical and electroretinographic study on activity of anthocyanosides. Arch Med Int 37:29-35, 1985
39. Wegmann R, Maeda K, Tronche P, and Bastide P: Effects of anthocyanosides on photoreceptors. Cytoenzymatic aspects. Ann Histochim 14:237-56, 1969
40. Stocker F: New ways of influencing the intraocular pressure. NY St J Med 49:58-63, 1949
41. Pautler EL and Ennis SR: The effect of diet on inherited retinal dystrophy in the rat. Curr Eye Res 3:1221-4, 1984
42. Hess H, Knapka JJ, Newsome DA, et al: Dietary prevention of cataracts in the pink-eyed RCS rat. Lag Anim Sci 35:47-53, 1985
43. Pautler EL, Maga JA and Tengerdy C: A pharmacologically potent natural product in the bovine retina. Exp Eye Res 42:285-8, 1986
44. Scharrer A and Ober M: Anthocyanosides in the treatment of retinopathies. Klin Monatsbl Augenheilkd 178:386-9, 1981
45. Sevin R and Cuendet JF: Effect of a combination of myrtillus anthocyanosides and beta-carotene on capillary resistance in diabetes. Ophthalmologica 152:109-17, 1966
46. Bever B and Zahnd G: Plants with oral hypoglycemic action. Quart J Crude Drug Res 17:139-96, 1979
47. Chaundry PS, Cambera J, Juliana HR, and Varma SD: Inhibition of human lens aldose reductase by flavonoids, sulindac and indomethacin. Biochem Pharmacol 32:1995-8, 1983
48. Varma SD, Mizuno A and Kinoshita JH: Diabetic cataracts and flavonoids. Science 195:87-9, 1977
49. Varma SD, El-aguizy HK and Richards RD: Refractive change in alloxan diabetic rabbits control by flavonoids I. Acta Ophthalmol 58:748-59, 1980
50. Allen FM: Blueberry leaf extract: Physiologic and clinical properties in relation to carbohydrate metabolism. JAMA 89:1577-81, 1927
51. Passariello N, Bisesti V and Sgambato S: Influence of anthocyanosides on the microcirculation and lipid picture in diabetic and dyslipidic subjects. Gazz Med Ital 138:563-6, 1979
52. Kadar A, Robert L, Miskulin M, et al: Influence of anthocyanoside treatment on the cholesterol-induced atherosclerosis in the rabbit. Paroi Arterielle 5:187-206, 1979
53. Coget J and Merlen JF: Clinical study of a new chemical agent for vascular protection. Difrarel 20, composed of anthocyanosides extracted from Vaccinium myrtillus. Phlebologie 21:221-8, 1968
54. Spinella G: Natural anthocyanosides in treatment of peripheral venous insufficiency. Arch Med Int 37:21-9, 1985
55. Coget JM and Merlen JF: Anthocyanosides and microcirculation. J Mal Vasc 5:43-6, 1980
56. Neumann L: Long-term therapy of vascular permeability disorders using anthocyanosides. Munch Med Wochenschr 115:952-4, 1973

Glossary

Abortifacient A substance that induces abortion.

Abscess A localized collection of pus and liquefied tissue in a cavity.

Acetylcholine One of the chemicals that transmits impulses between nerves and between nerves and muscle cells.

Acrid A pungent, biting taste that causes irritation.

Acute Having a rapid onset, severe symptoms, and a short course; not chronic.

Adaptogen A substance that is safe, increases resistance to stress, and has a balancing effect on body functions.

Adjuvant A substance that enhances the effect of the medicinal agent or increases the antigenicity of a cancer cell.

Adrenaline A hormone secreted by the adrenal gland that produces the "fight or flight" response. Also called epinephrine.

Aldosterone A hormone secreted by the adrenal gland that causes the retention of sodium and water.

Alkaloids Naturally occurring amines (nitrogen-containing compounds), arising from heterocyclic and often complex structures, that display pharmacological activity. Their trivial names usually end in -ine. They are usually classified according to the chemical structure of their main nucleus: phenylalkylamines (ephedrine), pyridine (nicotine), tropine (atropine, cocaine), quinoline (quinine), isoquinolone (papaverine), phenanthrene (morphine), purine (caffeine), imidazole (pilocarpine), and indole (physostigmine, yohimbine).

Allopathy A term that describes the conventional method of medicine that combats disease by using substances and techniques specifically against the disease.

Alterative A substance that produces a balancing effect on a particular body function.

231

Amebiasis An intestinal infection characterized by severe diarrhea caused by the parasite *Entamoeba histolytica*.

Amino acids A group of nitrogen-containing chemical compounds that form the basic structural units of proteins.

Analgesic A substance that reduces the sensation of pain.

Androgen Hormones that stimulate male characteristics.

Anthelminthic A substance that causes the elimination of intestinal worms.

Anthocyanidin A particular class of flavonoids that gives plants, fruits, and flowers colors ranging from red to blue.

Antibody Proteins manufactured by the body that bind to antigens to neutralize, inhibit, or destroy the antigen.

Antidote A substance that neutralizes or counteracts the effects of a poison.

Antigen Any substance that when introduced into the body causes the formation of antibodies against it.

Antihypertensive Having a blood pressure lowering effect.

Antioxidant A compound that prevents free radical or oxidative damage.

Aphrodisiac A substance that increases sexual desire.

Artery A blood vessel that carries oxygen-rich blood away from the heart.

Atherosclerosis A process in which fatty substances (cholesterol and triglycerides) are deposited in the walls of medium to large arteries, eventually leading to blockage of the artery.

Atopy A predisposition to various allergic conditions, including eczema and asthma.

Astringent An agent that causes the contraction of tissue.

Autoimmune A process in which antibodies develop against the body's own tissues.

Balm A soothing or healing medicine applied to the skin.

Basal metabolic rate The rate of metabolism when the body is at rest.

Basophil A type of white blood cell that is involved in allergic reactions.

Benign A mild disorder that usually is not fatal.

Beta-carotene Also known as pro-vitamin A, a plant carotene that can be converted to two vitamin A molecules.

Beta cell The cells in the pancreas that manufacture insulin.

Bilirubin The breakdown product of the hemoglobin molecule of red blood cells.

Biopsy A diagnostic test in which tissue or cells are removed from the body for examination under a microscope.

Bleeding time The time required for the cessation of bleeding from a small skin puncture as a result of platelet disintegration and blood vessel constriction. Ranges from 1 to 4 minutes.

Blood-brain barrier A special barrier that prevents the passage of materials from the blood to the brain.

Blood pressure The force exerted by blood as it presses against and attempts to stretch blood vessels.

Bromelain The protein-digesting enzyme found in pineapple.

Bursa A sac or pouch that contains a special fluid that lubricates joints.

Bursitis Inflammation of a bursa.

Calorie A unit of heat. A nutritional calorie is the amount of heat needed to raise 1 kg of water 1°C.

Candida albicans A yeast common to the intestinal tract.

Candidiasis A complex medical syndrome produced by a chronic overgrowth of the yeast *Candida albicans*.

Carbohydrate Sugars and starches.

Carcinogen Any agent or substance capable of causing cancer.

Carcinogenesis The development of cancer caused by the actions of certain chemicals, viruses, or unknown factors on primarily normal cells.

Cardiac output The volume of blood pumped from the heart in one minute.

Cardiopulmonary Pertaining to the heart and lungs.

Cardiotonic A compound that tones and strengthens the heart.

Carminative A substance that promotes the elimination of intestinal gas.

Carotene Fat-soluble plant pigments, some of which can be converted into vitamin A by the body.

Cartilage A type of connective tissue that acts as a shock absorber at joint interfaces.

Cathartic A substance that stimulates the movement of the bowels, more powerfully than a laxative.

Cholagogue A compound that stimulates the contraction of the gallbladder.

Cholecystitis Inflammation of the gallbladder.

Cholelithiasis Gallstones.

Choleretic A compound that promotes the flow of bile.

Cholestasis The stagnation of bile within the liver.

Cholinergic Pertaining to the parasympathetic portion of the autonomic nervous system and the release of acetylcholine as a transmitter substance.

Chronic Long-term or frequently recurring.

Cirrhosis A severe disease of the liver characterized by the replacement of liver cells with scar tissue.

Coenzyme A necessary nonprotein component of an enzyme, usually a vitamin or mineral.

Cold sore A small skin blister located anywhere around the mouth and caused by the herpes simplex virus.

Colic Severe, spasmodic pain that occurs in waves of increasing intensity, reaching a peak, then abating for a short time before returning.

Colitis Inflammation of the colon, usually associated with diarrhea that contains blood and mucus.

Collagen   The protein that is the main component of connective tissue.

Compress   A pad of linen applied under pressure to an area of skin and held in place.

Congestive heart failure   Chronic disease that results when the heart is not capable of supplying the oxygen demands of the body.

Connective tissue   The type of tissue that performs the function of providing support, structure, and cellular cement to the body.

Contagious   A disease that can be transferred from one person to another by social contact, such as sharing the home or workplace.

Coronary artery disease   A condition that occurs when the heart receives an inadequate supply of blood and oxygen as a result of atherosclerosis.

Corticosteroid drugs   A group of drugs similar to the natural corticosteroid hormones and used predominately in the treatment of inflammation and to suppress the immune system.

Corticosteroid hormones   A group of hormones produced by the adrenal glands that control the body's use of nutrients and the excretion of salts and water in the urine.

Cushing's syndrome   A condition caused by a hypersecretion of cortisone and characterized by spindly legs, "moon face," "buffalo hump," abdominal obesity, flushed facial skin, and poor wound healing.

Cyst   An abnormal lump or swelling, filled with fluid or semisolid material, in any body organ or tissue.

Cystitis   Inflammation of the inner lining of the bladder. It is usually caused by a bacterial infection.

Decoctions   Teas prepared by boiling the botanical with water for a specified period of time, followed by straining or filtering.

Dehydration   Excessive loss of water from the body.

Dementia   Senility. Loss of mental function.

Demineralization   Loss of minerals from the bone.

Demulcent   A soothing substance to irritated mucous membranes.

Dermatitis   Inflammation of the skin, sometimes due to allergy.

Diastolic   The second number in a blood pressure reading. It is the measure of the pressure in the arteries during the relaxation phase of the heart beat.

Disaccharide   A sugar composed of two monosaccharide units.

Diuretic   A compound that causes increased urination.

Diverticuli   Saclike outpouchings of the wall of the colon.

Double-blind study   A way of controlling against experimental bias by ensuring that neither the researcher nor the subject know when an active agent or placebo is being used.

Dysfunction   Abnormal function.

Dysplasia   Any abnormality of growth.

Edema   Accumulation of fluid in tissues (swelling).

Eicosapentaenoic acid (EPA) A fatty acid found primarily in cold-water fish.

Electroencephalogram A machine that measures and records brain waves.

Elimination diet A diet that eliminates allergic foods.

Emetic A substance that induces vomiting.

Emulsify The dispersement of large fat globules into smaller, uniformly distributed particles.

Encephalitis Inflammation of the brain usually as a result of viral infection.

Endometrium The mucous membrane lining of the uterus.

Enteric-coated A special way of coating a tablet or capsule to ensure that it does not dissolve in the stomach, so it can reach the intestinal tract.

Enzymes An organic catalyst that speeds chemical reactions.

Epidemiology The study of the occurrence and distribution of diseases in human populations.

Epinephrine See **adrenaline**.

Epithelium The cells that cover the entire surface of the body and that line most of the internal organs.

Epstein-Barr virus The virus that causes infectious mononucleosis and that is associated with Burkitt's lymphoma and nasopharyngeal cancer.

Essential fatty acid Fatty acids that the body cannot manufacture—linoleic and linolenic acids.

Essential oils Also known as volatile oils, ethereal oils, or essences. They are usually complex mixtures of a wide variety of organic compounds (e.g., alcohols, ketones, phenols, acids, ethers, esters, aldehydes, and oxides) that evaporate when exposed to air. They generally represent the odoriferous principles of plants.

Estrogens Hormones that exert female characteristics.

Excretion The process of elimination of waste products from a cell, tissue, or the entire body.

Extracellular The space outside the cell composed of fluid.

Extracts Concentrated forms of natural products, obtained by treating crude materials containing these substances with a solvent and then removing the solvent completely or partially from the preparation. The most commonly used extracts are fluid extracts, solid extracts, powdered extracts, tinctures, and native extracts.

Exudate Escaping fluid or semifluid material that oozes from a space that may contain serum, pus, and cellular debris.

Faruncle Another name for a boil that involves a hair follicle.

Fibrin A white insoluble protein formed by the clotting of blood, which serves as the starting point for wound repair and scar formation.

Fibrinolysis The dissolution of fibrin or a blood clot by the action of enzymes that convert insoluble fibrin into soluble particles.

Flavonoid   A generic term for a group of flavone-containing compounds that are found widely in nature. They include many of the compounds that account for plant pigments (anthocyanins, anthoxanthins, apigenins, flavones, flavonols, bioflavonols, etc.). These plant pigments exert a wide variety of physiological effects in the human body.

Fluid extracts   These extracts are typically hydroalcohol solutions with a strength of one part solvent to one part herb. The alcohol content varies with each product. They are, in essence, concentrated tinctures.

Free radicals   Highly reactive molecules, characterized by an unpaired electron, that can bind to and destroy cellular compounds.

Gerontology   The study of aging.

Giardiasis   An infection of the small intestine caused by the protozoan (single-celled) *Giardia lamblia*.

Gingivitis   Inflammation of the gums.

Glaucoma   A condition in which the pressure of the fluid in the eye is so high that it causes damage.

Glucose   A monosaccharide that is found in the blood and that is one of the body's primary energy sources.

Gluten   One of the proteins in wheat and some other grains that gives dough its tough, elastic character.

Glycosides   Sugar-containing compounds composed of a glycone (sugar component) and an aglycone (nonsugar-containing component) that can be cleaved on hydrolysis. The glycone portion may be glucose, rhamnose, xylose, fructose, arabinose, or any other sugar. The aglycone portion can be any kind of compound—e.g., sterols, triterpenes, anthraquinones, hydroquinones, tannins, carotenoids, or anthocyanidins.

Goblet cell   A goblet-shaped cell that secretes mucus.

Ground substance   The thick, gel-like material in which the cell fiber and blood capillaries of cartilage, bone, and connective tissue are embedded.

Helper T cell   Lymphocytes that help in the immune response.

Hematocrit   An expression of the percentage of blood occupied by blood cells.

Hemorrhoids   Distended veins in the lining of the anus.

Hepatic   Pertaining to the liver.

Hepatomegaly   Enlargement of the liver.

Holistic medicine   A form of therapy aimed at treating the whole person, not just the part or parts in which symptoms occur.

Hormone   A secretion of an endocrine gland that controls and regulates body functions.

Hyperglycemia   High blood sugar.

Hypersecretion   Excessive secretion.

Hypertension   High blood pressure.

Hypochlorhydria   Insufficient gastric acid output.

Hypoglycemia   Low blood sugar.

Hypolipidemic   Elevations of cholesterol and triglycerides in the blood.

Hypotension   Low blood pressure.

Hypoxia   An inadequate suppy of oxygen.

Iatrogenic   Literally, "physician produced." This term can be applied to any medical condition, disease, or other adverse occurrence that results from medical treatment.

Idiopathic   Of unknown cause.

Immunoglobulins   Antibodies.

Incidence   The number of new cases of a disease that occurs during a given period (usually years) in a defined population.

Incontinence   The inability to control urination or defecation.

Infarction   Death to a localized area of tissue as a result of an inadequate supply of oxygen.

Infusions   Teas produced by steeping the botanical substance in hot water.

Insulin   A hormone secreted by the pancreas. This hormone lowers blood sugar levels.

Interferon   A potent immune-enhancing substance that is produced by the body's cells to fight off viral infection and cancer.

In vitro   Outside a living body and in an artificial environment.

In vivo   In a living body of an animal or plant.

Jaundice   A condition caused by elevation of bilirubin in the body and characterized by a yellowing of the skin.

Keratin   An insoluble protein found in hair, skin, and nails.

Lactase   An enzyme that breaks down lactose into the monosaccharides glucose and galactose.

Lactose   One of the sugars present in milk. It is a disaccharide.

Laxative   A substance that promotes the evacuation of the bowels.

Lesion   Any localized, abnormal change in tissue formation.

Lethargy   A feeling of tiredness, drowsiness, or lack of energy.

Leukocyte   A white blood cell.

Leukotrienes   Inflammatory compounds produced when oxygen interacts with polyunsaturated fatty acids.

Lipid   Fats, phospholipids, steroids, and prostaglandins.

Lipotropic   Promoting the flow of lipids to and from the liver.

Lymph   Fluid contained in lymphatic vessels, which flows through the lymphatic system to be returned to the blood.

Lymphocyte   A type of white blood cell found primarily in lymph nodes.

Malabsorption   Impaired absorption of nutrients most often a result of diarrhea.

Malaise   A vague feeling of being sick or of physical discomfort.

Malignant   A term used to describe a condition that tends to worsen and eventually causes death.

Mast cell   A cell found in many tissues of the body that contributes greatly to allergic and inflammatory processes by secreting histamine and other similar particles.

Menorrhagia   Excessive loss of blood during menstrual periods.

Menstrums   Solvents used for extraction (e.g. water, alcohol, or acetone).

Metabolism   A collective term for all of the chemical processes that take place in the body.

Metabolite   A product of a chemical reaction.

Metalloenzyme   An enzyme that contains a metal at its active site.

Microbe   A popular term for microorganism.

Microflora   The microbial inhabitants of a particular region—e.g., the colon.

Mites   Small, eight-legged animals, less than $\frac{1}{20}$ in. (1.2 mm) long, similar to tiny spiders.

Molecule   The smallest complete unit of a substance that can exist independently and still retain the characteristic properties of the substance.

Monoclonal antibodies   Genetically engineered antibodies specific for one particular antibody.

Monosaccharide   A simple, one-unit sugar, like fructose or glucose.

Mortality rate   The number of deaths per 100,000 of the population per year.

Mucosa   Another term for mucous membrane.

Mucous membrane   The soft, pink, tissue that lines most of the cavities and tubes in the body, including the respiratory tract, gastrointestinal tract, genitourinary tract, and eyelids. The mucous membranes secrete mucus.

Mucus   The slick, slimy fluid secreted by the mucous membranes. Mucus acts as a lubricant and mechanical protector of the mucous membranes.

Mycotoxins   Toxins from yeast and fungi.

Myelin sheath   A white fatty substance that surrounds nerve cells to aid in nerve impulse transmission.

Neoplasia   A medical term for a tumor formation, characterized by a progressive, abnormal replication of cells.

Neurofibrillary tangles   Clusters of degenerated nerves.

Neurotransmitters   Substances that modify or transmit nerve impulses.

Night blindness   The inability to see well in dim light or at night.

Nocturia   The disturbance of a person's sleep at night by the need to pass urine.

Oleoresins   Primarily, mixtures of resins and volatile oils. They either occur naturally or are made by extracting the oily and resinous materials from botanicals with organic solvents (e.g., hexane, acetone, ether, alcohol). The solvent is then removed under vacuum, leaving behind a viscous, semisolid extract, which is the oleoresin. Examples of prepared oleoresins are paprika, ginger, and capsicum.

Oligoantigenic diet   See elimination diet.

Otitis media   Acute infection of the middle ear.

Pancreatin   A special extract of pork pancreas.

Papain   The protein-digesting enzyme of papaya.

Parkinson's disease   A slowly progressive, degenerating nervous system disease characterized by resting tremor, pill rolling of the fingers, a masklike facial expression, shuffling gait, and muscle rigidity and weakness.

Pathogen   Any agent, particularly a microorganism, that causes disease.

Pathogenesis   The process by which a disease originates and develops, particularly the cellular and physiologic processes.

Peristalsis   Successive muscular contractions of the intestines, which moves food through the intestinal tract.

Physiology   The study of the functioning of the body including the physical and chemical processes of its cells, tissues, organs, and systems.

Physostigmine   A drug that blocks the breakdown of acetylcholine.

Phytoestrogen   Plant compounds that exert estrogen effects.

Placebo   An inert or inactive substance used to test the efficacy of another substance.

Polysaccharide   A molecule composed of many sugar molecules linked together.

Powdered extract   A solid extract that has been dried as a powder.

Prostaglandin   Hormone-like compounds manufactured from essential fatty acids.

Psychosomatic   Pertaining to the relationship between the mind and body. Commonly used to refer to those physiological disorders thought to be caused entirely or partly by psychological factors.

Putrefaction   The process of breaking down protein compounds by rotting.

Recommended Dietary Allowance (RDA)   Officially recommended amounts of various nutrients.

Resins   Complex oxidative products of terpenes that occur naturally as plant exudates or are prepared by alcohol extraction of botanicals that contain resinous particles.

Saccharide   A sugar molecule.

Saponins   Non-nitrogenous glycosides, typically with sterol or triterpenes as the aglycone, that possess the common property of foaming, or making suds, when strongly agitated in an aqueous solution.

Satiety   A feeling of fullness or gratification.

Saturated fat   A fat whose carbon atoms are bonded to the maximum number of hydogen atoms; found in animal products like meat, milk, dairy products, and eggs.

Sclerosis   The process of hardening or scarring.

Senile dementia   Mental deterioration associated with aging.

Slow reacting substance of anaphylaxis (SRSA)   A potent allergic mediator produced and released by mast cells.

Solid extracts   Extracts that have had all of the residual solvent or liquid removed.

Submucosa   The tissue just below the mucous membrane.

Suppressor T cell   Lymphocytes controlled by the thymus gland and suppressing the immune response.

Syndrome   A group of signs and symptoms that occur together in a pattern characteristic of a particular disease or abnormal condition.

T cell   A lymphocyte that is under the control of the thymus gland.

Tincture   Alcohol or hydro-alcohol solutions usually containing the active principles of botanicals in low concentrations. They are usually prepared by maceration, percolation or by dilution of their corresponding fluid or native extracts. The strengths of tinctures are typically 1:10 or 1:5. Alcohol content will vary.

Tonic   A substance that exerts a gentle strengthening effect on the body.

Trans-**fatty acid**   The type of fat found in margarine.

Uremia   The retention of urine by the body, and the presence of high levels of urine components in the blood.

Urinalysis   The analysis of urine.

Urticaria   Hives.

Vasoconstriction   The constriction of blood vessels.

Vasodilation   The dilation of blood vessels.

Vitamin   An essential compound necessary to act as a catalyst in normal processes of the body.

Western diet   A diet characteristic of Western societies, i.e., a diet high in fat, refined carbohydrate, and processed foods and low in dietary fiber.

Wheal   The characteristic lesion in hives; a small welt.

Index